Dupuytren Disease

Editors

STEVEN C. HAASE
KEVIN C. CHUNG

HAND CLINICS

www.hand.theclinics.com

Consulting Editor
KEVIN C. CHUNG

August 2018 • Volume 34 • Number 3

ELSEVIER

1600 John F. Kennedy Boulevard • Suite 1800 • Philadelphia, Pennsylvania, 19103-2899

http://www.theclinics.com

HAND CLINICS Volume 34, Number 3
August 2018 ISSN 0749-0712, ISBN-13: 978-0-323-61388-0

Editor: Lauren Boyle
Developmental Editor: Kristen Helm

Hand Clinics (ISSN 0749-0712) is published quarterly by Elsevier Inc., 360 Park Avenue South, New York, NY 10010-1710. Months of publication are February, May, August, and November. Business and Editorial Offices: 1600 John F. Kennedy Blvd., Ste. 1800, Philadelphia, PA 19103-2899. Customer Service Office: 3251 Riverport Lane, Maryland Heights, MO 63043. Periodicals postage paid at New York, NY and at additional mailing offices. Subscription price is $422.00 per year (domestic individuals), $772.00 per year (domestic institutions), $100.00 per year (domestic students/residents), $481.00 per year (Canadian individuals), $898.00 per year (Canadian institutions), $541.00 per year (international individuals), $898.00 per year (international institutions), and $256.00 per year (international and Canadian students/residents). Foreign air speed delivery is included in all *Clinics* subscription prices. All prices are subject to change without notice. **POSTMASTER:** Send address changes to *Hand Clinics*, Elsevier Health Sciences Division, Subscription Customer Service, 3251 Riverport Lane, Maryland Heights, MO 63043. Customer Service (orders, claims, online, change of address): Elsevier Health Sciences Division, Subscription **Customer Service, 3251 Riverport Lane, Maryland Heights, MO 63043. Tel: 1-800-654-2452 (U.S. and Canada); 314-447-8871 (outside U.S. and Canada). Fax: 314-447-8029. E-mail: journalscustomerservice-usa@elsevier.com (for print support); journalsonlinesupport-usa@elsevier.com (for online support).**

Reprints. For copies of 100 or more of articles in this publication, please contact the Commercial Reprints Department, Elsevier Inc., 360 Park Avenue South, New York, New York 10010-1710. Tel.: 212-633-3874; Fax: 212-633-3820; E-mail: reprints@ elsevier.com.

Hand Clinics is covered in *MEDLINE/PubMed (Index Medicus), Current Contents/Clinical Medicine, EMBASE/Excerpta Medica,* and *ISI/BIOMED.*

Contributors

CONSULTING EDITOR

KEVIN C. CHUNG, MD, MS
Chief of Hand Surgery, University of Michigan Health System, Charles B.G. de Nancrede Professor of Plastic Surgery and Orthopaedic Surgery, Assistant Dean for Faculty Affairs, Associate Director of Global REACH, University of Michigan Medical School, Ann Arbor, Michigan, USA

EDITORS

STEVEN C. HAASE, MD
Associate Professor of Plastic and Orthopaedic Surgery, University of Michigan Medical School, Ann Arbor, Michigan, USA

KEVIN C. CHUNG, MD, MS
Chief of Hand Surgery, University of Michigan Health System, Charles B.G. de Nancrede Professor of Plastic Surgery and Orthopaedic Surgery, Assistant Dean for Faculty Affairs, Associate Director of Global REACH, University of Michigan Medical School, Ann Arbor, Michigan, USA

AUTHORS

SHEWEIDIN AZIZ, MBBS, MRCS (Eng)
University Hospitals of Leicester NHS Trust, AToMS, Leicester, United Kingdom

MARIE A. BADALAMENTE, PhD
Professor, Department of Orthopaedics, T-18 Health Science Center, Stony Brook University Medical Center, Stony Brook, New York, USA

PAUL BINHAMMER, MD, MSc, FRCSC
Division of Plastic and Reconstructive Surgery, Sunnybrook Health Sciences Centre, Toronto, Ontario, Canada

KEVIN C. CHUNG, MD, MS
Chief of Hand Surgery, University of Michigan Health System, Charles B.G. de Nancrede Professor of Plastic Surgery and Orthopaedic Surgery, Assistant Dean for Faculty Affairs, Associate Director of Global REACH, University of Michigan Medical School, Ann Arbor, Michigan, USA

NICHOLAS E. CROSBY, MD
Partner, Indiana Hand to Shoulder Center, Indianapolis, Indiana, USA

ILSE DEGREEF, MD, PhD, EBHS
Professor and Surgeon in Chief, Department of Orthopedic Surgery–Hand Unit, University Hospitals Leuven, University of Leuven, Leuven, Belgium

JOSEPH J. DIAS, MBBS, FRCS (Eng), MD (Res)
Professor, University Hospitals of Leicester NHS Trust, AToMS, Leicester, United Kingdom

KYLE R. EBERLIN, MD
Assistant Professor of Surgery, Associate Director, MGH Hand Surgery Fellowship, MGH Site Director, Harvard Plastic Surgery Residency Program, Massachusetts General Hospital, Harvard Medical School, Boston, Massachusetts, USA

KATE E. ELZINGA, MD, FRCSC
Clinical Lecturer, Section of Plastic Surgery, University of Calgary, Calgary, Alberta, Canada

STEVEN C. HAASE, MD
Associate Professor of Plastic and Orthopaedic Surgery, University of Michigan Medical School, Ann Arbor, Michigan, USA

SANDIP HINDOCHA, MD, MPhil, MBChB, MRCS, BTEC (Laser), MFFLM, FRCS (plast)
Professor, Lead Consultant Plastic, Reconstructive, Aesthetic, Laser and Hand Surgeon, Plastic Surgery and Laser Centre, Bedford Hospital NHS Trust, Bedford, United Kingdom

STEVEN E.R. HOVIUS, MD, PhD
Department of Plastic, Reconstructive and Hand Surgery, Erasmus MC, Hand and Wrist Surgery, Xpert Clinic, Rotterdam, The Netherlands; Department of Plastic Surgery, Radboudumc, Nijmegen, The Netherlands

LAWRENCE C. HURST, MD
Professor and Chairman, Department of Orthopaedics, T-18 Health Science Center, Stony Brook University Medical Center, Stony Brook, New York, USA

FREDERICK THOMAS D. KAPLAN, MD
Fellowship Director, Indiana Hand to Shoulder Center, Indianapolis, Indiana, USA

JENNIFER S. KARGEL, MD
Assistant Professor, Department of Plastic Surgery, University of Texas Southwestern Medical Center, VA North Texas Health Care System, Dallas, Texas, USA

STEPHEN J. LEIBOVIC, MD, MS
Clinical Associate Professor, Department of Orthopedic Surgery, Division of Plastic and Reconstructive Surgery, Virginia Commonwealth University, Virginia Hand Center, Richmond, Virginia, USA

MICHAEL J. MORHART, MD, MS, FRCSC
Clinical Professor, Division of Plastic Surgery, University of Alberta, Edmonton, Alberta, Canada

CHAITANYA S. MUDGAL, MD, MS (Orth), MCh (Orth)
Associate Professor in Orthopaedic Surgery, Hand Surgery Service, Department of Orthopaedics, Yawkey Center, Massachusetts General Hospital, Harvard Medical School, Boston, Massachusetts, USA

CHRISTINA TURESSON, ROT, PhD
Departments of Hand Surgery, Plastic Surgery and Burns, Linköping University, Linköping, Sweden; Department of Social and Welfare Studies, Linköping University, Norrköping, Sweden

PAUL M.N. WERKER, MD, PhD, FEBOPRAS, FEBHS
Professor and Chief, Department of Plastic Surgery, University Medical Center Groningen, University of Groningen, Groningen, The Netherlands

ANDREW Y. ZHANG, MD
Associate Professor, Department of Plastic Surgery, University of Texas Southwestern Medical Center, Parkland Memorial Hospital, Dallas, Texas, USA

CHAO ZHOU, MD
Hand and Wrist Surgery, Xpert Clinic, Rotterdam, The Netherlands; Department of Plastic and Reconstructive Surgery, Maastricht University Medical Center, Maastricht, The Netherlands

Contents

> Dupuytren disease is a fibroproliferative condition affecting the hands of millions of patients worldwide. The hypothesis of pathogenesis involves genetic factors and internal factors. Recent genome-wide association studies have provided much needed evidence for the long-held belief of a strong genetic component to the pathogenesis of Dupuytren disease. Specifically, abnormal activation of the Wnt signaling pathway plays an important role. Regarding internal factors, microvascular angiopathy and ischemia have been shown to lead to activation of transforming growth factor-β1 and proliferation of myofibroblasts.

> Dupuytren disease (DD) is a benign, fibroproliferative disease of unknown cause. The disease predominantly affects the palms of the hands, causing permanent digital contracture of the affected digits. DD is a late-onset disease and is often progressive, irreversible, and bilateral. The disease has a significant impact on the health care economy. The mainstay of treatment of DD is surgical excision of diseased palmar fascia. There is evidence of genetic susceptibility. This article introduces the epidemiology of DD and examines the Dupuytren diathesis to highlight the importance of identifying clinical severity in relation to patient counseling and recurrence risk following treatment.

> Dupuytren disease causes nodules and thickened fascial cords in the hands of affected individuals. In this article, the author explains normal fascial anatomy of the hand and describes how it relates to the pathologic anatomy found in Dupuytren disease. Anatomic findings in diseased cords are described, with particular reference to dangers encountered in the treatment of this condition.

> Needle aponeurotomy is an effective, minimally invasive treatment for metacarpophalangeal and interphalangeal joint contractures caused by Dupuytren disease. Multiple joints and digits can be safely treated in 1 session. Needle

aponeurotomy is more cost-effective and has a significantly lower complication rate compared with open fasciectomy and collagenase injections. Recurrence rates are higher compared with open fasciectomy and collagenase injections. Patient satisfaction rates are high following needle aponeurotomy; the single clinic visit required and the minimal downtime after treatment are advantages unique to this procedure compared with other treatment modalities, including open fasciectomy, dermatofasciectomy, collagenase injections, and lipofilling.

Proof-of-principle, basic-science studies, using a rat-tail tendon model and surgically removed Dupuytren cords, began collagenase *Clostridium histolyticum* (CCH) development. Clinical studies in humans were then conducted, where the primary end point was reduction in contracture to within 0° to 5° of extension. Phase 2 studies, which confirmed the optimal dose of collagenase as 0.58 mg, showed injectable CCH reduced contractures in metacarpophalangeal and proximal interphalangeal joints to within 0° to 5° in many joints and was well tolerated. Clinical results from phase 3 studies confirmed the efficacy and safety of injectable CCH as a viable nonsurgical intervention.

This article discusses limited fasciectomy for Dupuytren contracture, reviews the literature to list common complications, addresses the observations that need to be made after surgery, and systematically reviews the literature for 2 clinical questions: (1) regarding leaving wounds open and (2) the use of postoperative splintage.

Clinicians struggle with limited efficacy and durability of standard treatments when treating patients with Dupuytren disease diathesis. Alternative treatments such as low-dose radiation therapy in the early phase of disease, supplemental pharmacotherapy with antiinflammatory and/or antimitotic drugs, as well as other pharmacologic targets, and more aggressive surgery such as dermofasciectomy all have been reported with variable success or with serious side effects that hamper their standard use. This article gives an overview of the available literature.

Despite more than a hundred years of publications on Dupuytren disease, there has been a lack of consensus on definitions and outcomes until recently. Staging and classifications systems have an important historical context; however, more recently, outcomes rely on patient-reported outcomes, angular correction, and definitions of recurrence. This article reviews commonly used assessments, classifications, and staging systems for Dupuytren disease.

Dupuytren contracture is a progressive disease involving collagen within the palmar fascia. When the contracture progresses to meet specific parameters, intervention is considered and includes collagenase injection, percutaneous or open fasciotomy, or palmar fasciectomy. Complications after treatment include contracture recurrence, digital nerve injury or postoperative neurapraxia, flexor tendon injury/rupture, delayed wound healing or skin necrosis, dysvascular digit/arterial injury, hematoma, and infection. Patients with severe or recurrent Dupuytren contracture are more likely to experience complications. Patient education is paramount; one must consider the patient's goals for treatment, functional requirements, time frame for recovery, and tolerance for complications when deciding about treatment.

The role of hand therapy in the treatment of Dupuytren disease varies depending on the patient and the procedure. There is limited evidence for hand therapy as a preventive treatment of Dupuytren disease. Before corrective treatment, the hand therapist can contribute with assessments to promote evaluation of outcome. After corrective treatment, hand therapy is tailored to each patient's needs and consists of orthoses, exercise, edema control, and pain or scar management. Orthoses are usually part of the hand therapy protocol after corrective procedures despite lack of strong supporting evidence and should be provided based on individual patient needs.

 Video content accompanies this article at http://www.hand.theclinics.com.

Treatment of recurrent Dupuytren disease is challenging. Multiple options exist, each having relative benefits and weaknesses. Choice for optimal treatment is made on a case-by-case basis, with shared decision-making with the patient. Percutaneous and enzymatic techniques are best reserved for patients with well-defined recurrent disease and offer the benefit of quicker recovery with minimal or no scarring. Surgical treatments have higher risks of neurovascular injury and scarring but lower recurrence rates. Staged continuous passive elongation followed by dermofasciectomy may lower neurovascular injury and improve outcomes. Salvage procedures may be necessary in patients with poor tissue beds and neurovascular compromise.

A comparison is provided between minimally invasive techniques and limited fasciectomy (LF) in the treatment of Dupuytren disease. A technique called percutaneous needle aponeurotomy and lipofilling is described. In a randomized controlled trial, there is no significant difference between this technique and LF after 1 year in contracture correction and recurrent contractures. At 5 years post operation, however, there is a significant change in recurrence rates in favor of LF. Patients with moderate diathesis should choose between minimally invasive technique with early recurrence, fast recovery, and few complications versus late recurrence, slower recovery, and more complications, as observed with LF or dermofasciectomy.

As minimally invasive options for treatment of Dupuytren contractures become increasingly widespread, it is important that the evidence is carefully evaluated and patients are informed of the risks and benefits of the options available. The authors advocate a shared decision-making process, using evidence-based medicine, to guide patients in their treatment choices. In this article, the authors present their thoughtful approach to selecting the appropriate Dupuytren treatment of patients, along with detailed, practical technical tips to avoid complications during the execution of these interventions; both collagenase injection and limited fasciectomy techniques are described in detail.

HAND CLINICS

THE CLINICS ARE AVAILABLE ONLINE!
Access your subscription at:
www.theclinics.com

Preface
Dupuytren Disease

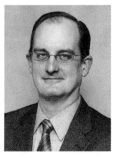 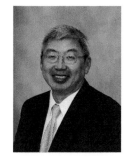

Steven C. Haase, MD   Kevin C. Chung, MD, MS

Editors

In business, "disruptive technology" quickly changes the landscape of how consumers embrace new products to improve their quality of life. For example, smart phones now help us to connect with everyone around the world. Mass distribution of quality products from Costco has propelled a new business model of direct-consumer marketing. In medicine, complex surgical treatment of Dupuytren contracture has been the mainstay of treatment, but the application of collagenase and needle aponeurotomy techniques are becoming more prevalent and are establishing their place as suitable options for this disease. Although initially viewed by some as "disruptive," one could argue that these minimally invasive techniques should now be labeled as "sustaining technology."

Associated with these new treatment options is the uncertainty that physicians and patients often have in choosing the appropriate treatments. The concepts of shared decision making, patient-centered care, and evidence-based medicine ought to be applied in guiding physicians to provide the best value for patients. Patients need the most up-to-date data to make an informed judgment regarding outcomes and cost associated with these techniques. After careful consideration of the options, the patient and the surgeon commit to a most judicious treatment course.

This *Hand Clinics* issue is devoted to such an approach by presenting treatment data and sharing techniques from authorities in the field. Authors from various regions of the world share their guidance and their treatment approaches on this common condition that still defies a cause after its description over 200 years ago. We appreciated their contributions that serve as a benchmark for all of us in treating this condition. The final article from us provides a personalized treatment approach in managing this condition at the University of Michigan. We describe the step-by-step approach for collagenase injection and for fasciectomy to achieve the most predictable outcomes in our hands. We have strived to organize an authoritative issue that can be helpful in delivering information in a concise fashion.

We are grateful for your continued interest in *Hand Clinics*. Please do feel free to share topics that you feel should be presented in future issues.

Steven C. Haase, MD
University of Michigan Medical School
2130 Taubman Center
1500 East Medical Center Drive
Ann Arbor, MI 48109-0340, USA

Kevin C. Chung, MD, MS
Michigan Medicine
University of Michigan Medical School
2130 Taubman Center
1500 East Medical Center Drive
Ann Arbor, MI 48109-0340, USA

E-mail addresses:
shaase@med.umich.edu (S.C. Haase)
kecchung@med.umich.edu (K.C. Chung)

Hand Clin 34 (2018) xi
https://doi.org/10.1016/j.hcl.2018.04.004
0749-0712/18/© 2018 Published by Elsevier Inc.

Errata

A few errors were made in the August 2017 issue of *Hand Clinics* (Volume 33, Issue 3) in the article, "Mobilization of Joints of the Hand with Symphalangism," by Goo Hyun Baek, Jihyeung Kim, and Jin Woo Park. The Figure 6 legend on page 555 should read, "Two and a half years after the operation, left index PIP joint was fused (second from left) but the third PIP joint (first from right) maintained joint space and congruity." Under the Outcomes section on page 558, the authors operated on "7 thumb IP joints (5 patients; 3 boys and 2 girls)." The last two sentences on this page should read, "The mean gain of active flexion in the remaining 58 joints was 65° (range 20°–100°). The duration of follow-up was a mean of 2.8 (range 1–12) years." The online version of the article has been corrected.

In the May 2018 issue of *Hand Clinics* (Volume 34, Issue 2), the affiliations for Scott Wolfe and Elizabeth Inkellis are listed incorrectly. The affiliations for both authors are:

Scott W. Wolfe, MD
Chief Emeritus, Hand and Upper Extremity Surgery
Hospital for Special Surgery
Professor of Orthopedic Surgery
Weill Medical College of Cornell University
New York, New York, USA

Elizabeth Inkellis, MD
Hand and Upper Extremity Surgery
Hospital for Special Surgery
Weill Medical College of Cornell University
New York, New York, USA

The online version of this issue has been corrected.

Hand Clin 34 (2018) xiii
https://doi.org/10.1016/j.hcl.2018.05.001

The Basic Science of Dupuytren Disease

Andrew Y. Zhang, MD[a],*, Jennifer S. Kargel, MD[b]

KEYWORDS

- Dupuytren disease • Pathogenesis • Genetics • Myofibroblast • Wnt pathway • Growth factors

KEY POINTS

- Proliferation of myofibroblasts leads to shortening of Dupuytren disease cord resulting in flexion contracture of the finger.
- The transformation of fibroblasts into myofibroblasts and the force transduction involving α-actin are mediated by many cytokines, including TGF-β, PDGF, and IL-1.
- Based on recent studies, the Wnt pathway and transcription factor MafB play important roles in the pathogenesis of Dupuytren disease.

PATHOPHYSIOLOGY

The pathophysiology of Dupuytren disease (DD) is centered around myofibroblasts.[1] These cells originate as fibroblasts that make collagen and have intracytoplasmic myofibrillar bundles that are able to contract, contributing to the progressive shortening of cords, which in turn leads to soft tissue and joint contractures.

The progression of DD is divided into three stages, originally described by Luck[2] in 1959. During the first stage, proliferation, fibroblasts proliferate and nodules develop. In the second involutional stage, these fibroblasts are upregulated and transformed into myofibroblasts, which align with lines of stress in the hand that pass through the nodules. Type III collagen is deposited, and this connective tissue begins to organize and develop into cords, which then start to contract. There is a relative overabundance of type III collagen because of increased density of fibroblasts and decreased production of the "normal" type I collagen. The final stage is called the residual stage, in which the nodules regress, and the cords become hypocellular and scarlike, causing further contracture development.

In each phase, multiple factors contribute to this pathologic process. Genetics plays a vital role, as do internal factors, such as activation of growth factors, cytokines, and free radicals.

GENETIC FACTORS

DD has a prevalence of 0.5% to 11% of the general population, and most commonly affects men of northern European heritage.[3] The condition usually presents after the age of 50 and is often bilateral. It is a familial disorder with a strong genetic predisposition and likely variable autosomal-dominant pattern of inheritance,[3] although to date there is no way to test for DD using genetic testing.

No single gene has been identified as the primary cause, although certain genetic mutations may lead to and contribute to the severity of disease. Ojwang and colleagues[4] suggested that it has a complex multifactorial cause. In their 2010 study, they performed genome-wide association scans to search for regions on the genome that may have a role in DD, identifying associated regions in chromosomes 6, 11, and 16.

Financial Disclosure: The authors have no commercial or financial conflicts of interests to declare.
[a] Department of Plastic Surgery, University of Texas Southwestern Medical Center, 1801 Inwood Road, Dallas, TX 75390-1932, USA; [b] Department of Plastic Surgery, University of Texas Southwestern Medical Center, VA North Texas Health Care System, 4500 S. Lancaster Road, Dallas, TX 75216, USA
* Corresponding author.
E-mail address: Dr.zhang@gmail.com

Bayat and colleagues[5] identified a group of patients with a maternally transmitted inheritance pattern of DD. This cohort was found to have a mitochondrial genome mutation involving the mitochondrial 16s ribosomal RNA region, resulting in free radical generation and defective apoptosis in the Dupuytren tissue.

When the disease process is activated, multiple genes are upregulated to begin myofibroblastic proliferation, including transforming growth factor (TGF)-β messenger RNA expression.[6] More than 20 unique genes were found to be significantly upregulated in a microarray analysis by Zhang and colleagues.[7] Many of the upregulated genes have been previously shown to be involved in DD pathogenesis. These include α-smooth muscle actin, fibronectin, β1 integrin, laminin, tanascin C, Hsp47, TGF-β2, and collagen type I. Several significantly upregulated genes that had not been previously characterized were collagen type V, α-2 (COL5A2), collagen type VIII, α-1 (COL8A1), contactin I (CNTN1), leucine-rich repeat containing 17 (LRRC17), and musculoaponeurotic fibrosarcoma oncogene homolog B or MafB. In another study by the same authors, MafB, which showed a four-fold increase in

Dupuyten cord tissue, was shown to be localized within cells containing α-smooth muscle actin (a marker of myofibroblasts).[8]

The Maf oncogene was initially identified in an oncogenic avian retrovirus that induced musculoaponeurotic fibrosarcomas in vivo and cellular transformation of fibroblasts when expressed in chicken embryos in vitro. The origin of the family name Maf is taken from musculoaponeurotic fibrosarcoma.[9] DD in its early stages is histopathologically similar to fibrosarcoma.[10] This ability to cause transformation of fibroblasts makes MafB relevant to the pathogenesis of DD.

Wnt signaling pathways have recently been strongly implicated in the pathogenesis of DD.[11] The Wnt gene family consists of structurally related genes that encode glycoproteins, which are extracellular signaling molecules. Abnormal Wnt signaling is linked to a range of diseases, most notably cancer. The best-understood Wnt signaling pathway is the canonical pathway, which activates the nuclear functions of β-catenin, leading to changes in gene expression that influence cell proliferation and survival (**Fig. 1**).[12] β-catenin has been shown to be present in increased concentration in DD cord tissue.[13] In a study

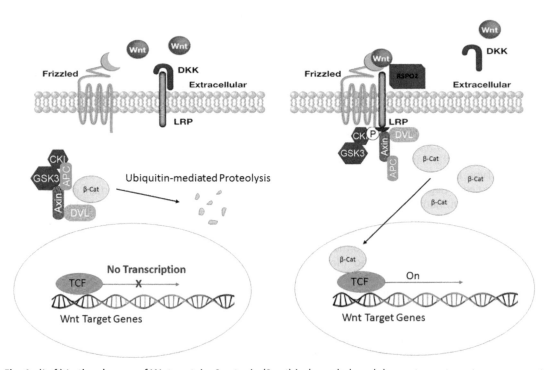

Fig. 1. (*Left*) In the absence of Wnt protein, β-catenin (β-cat) is degraded, and down-stream target genes are not activated. (*Right*) If Wnt signaling is active, β-cat degradation is reduced. R-spondin (RSPO2) positively regulates β-cat signaling by interacting with the Frizzled receptor and the low-density lipoprotein-receptor-related protein (LRP) and by competing with the dickkopf protein (DKK) for LRP. APC, adenomatous polyposis coli protein; Axin, AXIN1, a cytoplasmic protein; CK1, casein kinase 1; DVL, disheveled protein; GSK3, glycogen synthase kinase 3; P, phosphorylation; TCF, T-cell factor.

comparing the genomes of more than 2000 patients with DD compared with more than 11,000 control subjects, Dolmans and colleagues[11] found nine chromosomal loci associated with DD, six of which contained genes in the Wnt signaling pathway: WNT2, WNT4, SFRP4, SULF1, WNT7B, and RSPO2. Interestingly, the three remaining upregulated loci that lack an obvious connection to the Wnt pathway are related to the MafB gene.

A meta-analysis of genome-wide association scans studies confirmed the findings of Dolmans and colleagues[11] and found further evidence of Wnt signaling pathway's involvement in DD.[14] Another study showed that at least a proportion of DD sufferers may have reduced or absent expression of several microRNAs that restrain the Wnt pathway through lack of regulation of genes, such as WNT5A, ZIC1, and TGFB1.[15]

INTERNAL FACTORS

Early analysis concentrated on the roles of ischemia and free radicals in the development of DD.[16,17] Microangiopathy and ischemia of the palmar fascia can occur following trauma. Vessels in the diseased fascia of patients with DD are surrounded by fibroblasts and lined with many layers of basal laminae, resulting in relative narrowing of the vessel. As trauma leads to release of cytokines and upregulation of fibroblasts, localized ischemia develops and adenosine triphosphate is broken down to hypoxanthine and xanthine. Xanthine dehydrogenase is converted to its more toxic form xanthine oxidase and releases superoxide free radicals. The free radicals then stimulate further fibroblast proliferation and production of cytokines. This results in additional thickening of the vessels because of the higher concentration of surrounding fibroblasts with subsequent decreased blood flow and ischemia.

The focus has now shifted to better understanding the mechanotransduction and cell/extracellular matrix interaction mediated by cytokine production and activation. It is believed that these mechanosignaling processes, in which cells sense mechanical forces and then change their intracellular biochemistry and gene expression, are the driving forces behind the disease. Eaton[18] describes this process as a reactive overresponse to mechanical forces at a cellular level.

The cytokine TGF-β is upregulated in Dupuytren tissues and is believed to be the main growth factor involved in the disease process, as evidenced by increased production of and increased sensitivity of the implicated cells to this molecule. TGF-β regulates the transcription of a wide spectrum of matrix proteins including collagen, fibronectin, glycosaminoglycans, matrix-degrading proteases and their inhibitors, and integrin receptors.[19] Many of these proteins have been found to be abnormal in DD. TGF-β is released from many cell types that are involved in inflammation and fibrosis, including lymphocytes, macrophages, endothelial cells, smooth muscle cells, epithelial cells, and fibroblasts.

There are three mammalian isoforms of TGF-β: TGF-β1, TGF-β2, and TGF-β3. These TGF-β isoforms have been identified in the fibroblastic nodule and surrounding tissue of DD palmar fascia. Using real-time polymerase chain reaction (a method to detect the expression of the messenger RNA for a protein), Baird and colleagues[20] found increased TGF-β expression in DD. TGF-β isoforms, however, were not distinguished in this study. In a later study, Berndt and colleagues[21] identified all three TGF-β isoforms in DD cord tissue, and TGF-β1 and -β3 were also found in the surrounding tissue using in situ hybridization (a method to detect specific protein expression in tissue sections). Badalamente and colleagues[22] demonstrated TGF-β1 staining in fibroblasts, myofibroblasts, and capillary endothelial cells in DD samples, whereas TGF-β2 was found only in myofibroblasts.

TGF-β induces differentiation of fibroblasts into myofibroblasts and stimulation of these cells to produce collagen. Although normal palmar fascia is composed of principally type I collagen, DD cords have increased type III collagen, resulting in a larger ratio of type III to type I. This is directly related to fibroblast density: fibroblasts preferentially reduce their production of type I collagen when their density is increased.[23] The stimulation of these cells by growth factors to continue to produce collagen leads to an increase in type III collagen, decreased apoptosis of fibroblasts, and an imbalance between collagenases and their inhibitors.[17]

Another important growth factor seen in DD is platelet-derived growth factor (PDGF), which is associated with myofibroblasts in the hypercellular proliferative phase. Once bound to cell membrane surface receptors, PDGF activates intracellular activities including increased protein synthesis, increased type III collagen production, and reorganization of actin filaments. It also acts synergistically with other growth factors to stimulate cell proliferation.[24,25]

Additional growth factors and cytokines upregulated in DD include fibroblast growth factor, TGF-α, epidermal growth factor, and interleukin (IL)-1.[17] The cytokine IL-1 is the most abundant cytokine in DD tissue, stimulating platelets and macrophages to produce growth factors, inducing expression of transcriptional factors to cause fibroblast proliferation, and signaling Langerhans cells to migrate to the dermoepidermal junction and DD nodules.

Once activated, the myofibroblasts have large intracellular bundles of α-smooth muscle actin microfilaments that align within the cells and extend to the cellular membrane.[26] The greatest percentage of fibroblasts with these bundles is found in the proliferative stage; the expression decreases slightly in the involutional stage and is nearly absent in the residual stage.[27]

These α-smooth muscle actin bundles then develop a transmembranous connection through integrins with adjacent extracellular filamentous complexes made of fine fibrils of fibronectin that are 3 to 5 nm in diameter and some larger fibrils measuring 10 to 13 nm in diameter.[28] The fibronectin complex has multiple domains that can bind to the surface of the cells and to the surrounding collagen. Once the intracellular contractile force is generated, it is transmitted into the surrounding tissue via these extracellular fibronectin complexes, which in turn leads to tissue contracture.

Understanding of the basic science of DD has increased dramatically over the last 50 years. Although the exact cause of the disease still remains a mystery, and there are no current genetic tests for DD, it is now known that certain key genes, such as MafB and the Wnt signaling pathway, are involved and that transformation of fibroblasts into myofibroblasts is a key component of the disease. Within the myofibroblasts, α-smooth muscle actin bundles interact with extracellular fibonectin complexes to transmit contractile forces to the surrounding tissues. During this process, cytokines, such as TGF-β, PDGF, and IL-1, are activated and stimulate cell proliferation and migration, release of growth factors, and further production of collagen. As understanding of this disease unfolds on a cellular level, future areas of study will likely focus on gene-targeted therapy and cytokine-level pharmacologic interventions to treat this disease in a more minimally invasive fashion.

REFERENCES

1. Gabbiani G, Majno G. Dupuytren's contracture: fibroblast contraction? An ultrastructural study. Am J Pathol 1972;66:131–46.
2. Luck JV. Dupuytren's contracture: a new concept of the pathogenesis correlated with surgical management. J Bone Joint Surg Am 1959;41-A(4):635–64.
3. DiBenedetti DB, Nguyen D, Zografos L, et al. Prevalence, incidence, and treatments of Dupuytren's disease in the United States: results from a population-based study. Hand (N Y) 2011;6(2):149–58.
4. Ojwang JO, Adrianto I, Gray-McGuire C, et al. Genome-wide association scan of Dupuytren's disease. J Hand Surg Am 2010;35:2039–45.
5. Bayat A, Walter J, Lambe H, et al. Identification of a novel mitochondrial mutation in Dupuytren's disease using multiplex DHPLC. Plast Reconstr Surg 2005;115:134–41.
6. Bayat A, Watson JS, Stanley JK, et al. Genetic susceptibility to Dupuytren disease: association of Zf9 transcription factor gene. Plast Reconstr Surg 2003;111:2133–9.
7. Zhang AY, Fong KD, Pham H, et al. Gene expression analysis of Dupuytren's disease: the role of TGF beta2. J Hand Surg Eur Vol 2008;33(6):783–90.
8. Lee L, Zhang AY, Chong A, et al. Expression of a novel gene, MafB, in Dupuytren's disease. J Hand Surg Am 2006;31:211–8.
9. Nishizawa M, Kataoka K, Goto N, et al. v-maf, a viral oncogene that encodes a "leucine zipper" motif. Proc Natl Acad Sci U S A 1989;86:7711–5.
10. Erdmann MW, Quaba AA, Sommerlad BC. Epithelioid sarcoma masquerading as Dupuytren's disease. Br J Plast Surg 1995;48:39–42.
11. Dolmans GH, Werker PM, Hennies HC, et al. Wnt signaling and Dupuytren's disease. N Engl J Med 2011;365(4):307–17.
12. Moon RT, Kohn AD, De Ferrari GV, et al. WNT and beta-catenin signaling: diseases and therapies. Nat Rev Genet 2004;5:691–701.
13. Varallo VM, Gan BS, Seney S, et al. Betacatenin expression in Dupuytren's disease: potential role for cell-matrix interactions in modulating beta-catenin levels in vivo and in vitro. Oncogene 2003;22(24):3680–4.
14. Becker K, Siegert S, Toliat MR, et al. Meta-analysis of genome-wide association studies and network analysis-based integration with gene expression data identify new suggestive loci and unravel a Wnt-centric network associated with Dupuytren's disease. PLoS One 2016;11(7):e0158101.
15. Mosakhani N, Guled M, Lahti L, et al. Unique microRNA profile in Dupuytren's contracture supports deregulation of beta-catenin pathway. Mod Pathol 2010;23(11):1544–52.
16. Murrell GAC. Scientific comment: basic science of Dupuytren's disease. Ann Chir Main Memb Super 1992;11(5):355–61.
17. Al-Qattan MM. Factors in the pathogenesis of Dupuytren's contracture. J Hand Surg Am 2006;31:1527–34.
18. Eaton C. Evidence-based medicine: Dupuytren contracture. Plast Reconstr Surg 2014;133:1241–51.

19. Roberts AB, Sporn MB. Transforming growth factor-b. In: Clark RAF, editor. The molecular and cellular biology of wound repair. 2nd edition. New York: Plenum Press; 1995. p. 275–308.

20. Baird KS, Crossan JF, Ralston SH. Abnormal growth factor and cytokine expression in Dupuytren's contracture. J Clin Pathol 1993;46:425–8.

21. Berndt A, Kosmehl H, Mandel U, et al. TGF beta and bFGF synthesis and localization in Dupuytren's disease (nodular palmar fibromatosis) relative to cellular activity, myofibroblast phenotype and onco-fetal variants of fibronectin. Histochem J 1995;27:1014–20.

22. Badalamente MA, Sampson SP, Hurst LC, et al. The role of transforming growth factor beta in Dupuytren's disease. J Hand Surg Am 1996;21:210–5.

23. Murrell GAC, Francis MJO, Bromley L. The collagen changes of Dupuytren's contracture. J Hand Surg Br 1991;16:263–6.

24. Badalamente M, Hurst L, Grandia S, et al. Platelet-derived growth factor in Dupuytren's disease. J Hand Surg Am 1992;17(2):317–23.

25. Terek R, Jiranek W, Goldberg M, et al. The expression of platelet-derived growth-factor gene in Dupuytren contracture. J Bone Joint Surg Am 1995;77:1–9.

26. Tomasek JJ, Gabbiani G, Hinz B, et al. Myofibroblasts and mechano-regulation of connective tissue remodeling. Nat Rev Mol Cell Biol 2002;3:349–63.

27. Tomasek JJ, Rayan GM. Correlation of α-smooth muscle actin expression and contraction in Dupuytren's disease fibroblasts. J Hand Surg Am 1995;20:450–5.

28. Tomasek JJ, Schultz RJ, Haaksma CJ. Extracellular matrix-cytoskeletal connections at the surface of the specialized contractile fibroblast (myofibroblast) in Dupuytren disease. J Bone Joint Surg Am 1987;69:1400–7.

Risk Factors, Disease Associations, and Dupuytren Diathesis

Sandip Hindocha, MD, MPhil, MBChB, MRCS, BTEC(Laser), MFFLM, FRCS(plast)

KEYWORDS

- Dupuytren disease • Epidemiology • Risk factors • Diathesis • Inheritance

KEY POINTS

- Dupuytren disease (DD) is most prevalent in the northern European population and is reported less frequently in other geographic areas.
- Cases of DD in non-European populations likely reflect migration patterns.
- Several risk factors have been found to be associated with DD.
- DD is a heritable condition; although many studies identify an inheritance pattern of autosomal dominance with variable penetrance, more recent studies have shown it to be a multifactorial and polygenic condition.

INTRODUCTION AND OVERVIEW OF THE EPIDEMIOLOGY OF DUPUYTREN DISEASE

Dupuytren disease (DD) has been recognized for several centuries; it was first described as a medical condition by Plater of Basle in 1614.[1,2] Even though its pathogenesis remains largely unknown, the epidemiology of DD has been studied extensively.[3–6]

Globally, the prevalence of DD varies from 3% to 42%[3] (**Fig. 1**). A geographic imbalance has been described in the distribution of DD. The disease seems to be most prevalent in northern European white people,[7] where it is one of the most common inherited connective tissue disorders. Its prevalence has been reported to reach up to 30% in the Norwegian population aged more than 60 years.[8,9] Furthermore, a prevalence of 9.4% in men and 2.8% in women has been described from Norway,[9] and a prevalence of 13.3% was reported in an Icelandic study.[10] Although the European prevalence is generally higher in northern compared with Mediterranean countries,[3] a fairly high prevalence has been reported in Spain.[11] No other studies have been found from southern Europe. The familial incidence has been reported to be 44% and 74%, respectively, in populations from Sweden and Iceland.[4,12]

By contrast, the prevalence rate of DD is reported to be slightly more than 4% in the male population in England.[8] In Germany, the prevalence of DD has been estimated to be 2.5%.[13] In a comparison of prevalence rates in studies from various countries worldwide, the mean prevalence was reported as less than 5%, and was similar in men and women in persons up to 45 years of age. It increases to 33% in men older than 65 years and 23% in women older than 75 years.[14]

Contrary to the findings of previous studies, a high prevalence of DD has been noted in a recent study in Bosnia and Herzegovina.[15] Most cases had only palmar changes; those individuals with moderate contracture may not have sought medical attention where the health economy was struggling in a postwar era, suggesting under-reporting and a lower than predicted prevalence rate. Ethnic differences in Bosnia (Serbian Croat and Muslim Croat) in the prevalence of DD have been documented in Bosnia,[15] and this may suggest

Plastic Surgery & Laser Centre, Bedford Hospital NHS Trust, Reception J, Kempston Road, Bedford MK429DJ, UK
E-mail address: sandiphindocha@gmail.com

Hand Clin 34 (2018) 307–314
https://doi.org/10.1016/j.hcl.2018.03.002

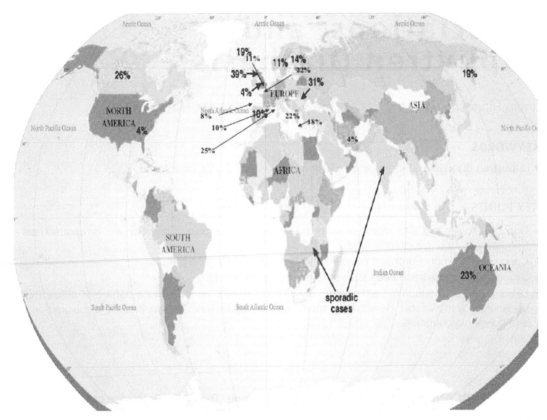

Fig. 1. Global distribution of DD. (*From* Hindocha S, McGrouther DA, Bayat A. Epidemiological evaluation of Dupuytren's disease incidence and prevalence rates in relation to etiology. Hand (N Y) 2009; 4(3):262; with permission.)

migratory changes over the years with the possibility of the Serbian Croat population migrating from northern European ancestry.[16]

Similarly, in Norway, ethnic differences in the prevalence of DD after the age of 60 years is noted. Prevalence of DD in the Norwegian community is greater compared with that of the Sami population but this difference is not significant, suggesting a mixture of genetic and environmental factors. In the United Kingdom it seems that prevalence is much higher in Scotland (>30% in the >60 years age group)[14] compared with England (4%).[8] Such a varying prevalence suggests a migratory pattern of DD from northern Europe.[16] DD is frequently labeled as the Viking or Nordic disease. However, other than the high prevalence of DD in Scandinavia, there has been no concrete evidence to date that supports the Nordic origin of the disease.[17] These studies should be compared with caution. Although they represent prevalence of DD in various populations, methodologies of data collection, age categorization of patients, and experience of examiners collecting data is extremely variable.

Importantly, not all cases of DD can be easily attributed to migration of a northern European disease. There are several reports of cases of DD around the world where the disease would not be expected to be found based on migration alone, such as the African or Asian continents. For example, DD has been identified in nonwhite, non-European patients identified on the African continent.[18–25] In addition, the disease has been reported in Asia.[26–30] None of the individual cases reported in Africa or Asia had a positive family history, which argues against a migrating population, and suggests environmental factors may play a role. Risk factors and disease associations with DD are explored next.

RISK FACTORS AND DISEASE ASSOCIATIONS OF DUPUYTREN DISEASE

The heritable nature of DD has been of great interest, with reports of the disease present in as many as 3 generations[31] and studies suggesting a possible autosomal dominant inheritance pattern.[32] However, it is possible that the multifactorial cause of DD also includes a strong environmental factor based on the results of Finsen and colleagues,[33] who found that family members were more likely to develop DD if they were residing in the same geographic area as their diseased relative. Several studies have shown support for an environmental influence in the development of DD, as highlighted in **Table 1**.

Risk factors associated with DD are summarized in **Box 1**. Each is reviewed in detail later.

Age-Specific Epidemiology of Dupuytren Disease

Prevalence rates of DD range from 0.2% to 56% in varying age groups and depend on methods of data collection. The prevalence of DD increases with age, with a mean age of onset of 49 years in patients with a positive family history.[34] Increasing prevalence with age argues for an environmental exposure that accumulates over time, although, in cases with a known family background for DD, the onset tends to be earlier and the course of the disease more severe.

DD in the younger population is more likely to have a genetic predisposition than some environmental influence.[35–37] The differential diagnosis of a child who presents with a nodule in the hand, contracture of a digit, or a knuckle pad on the dorsum of the hand would not typically include

DD, but it has been reported.[38] Therefore, DD should be included in the differential diagnosis, especially if the patient is of northern European descent.[34] A nonfamilial, sporadic case of DD has been identified in a child as young as 6 months old,[39] which strongly supports the genetic nature of the disease.

Gender-Specific Epidemiology of Dupuytren Disease

Early literature stated that DD did not occur in women.[40] However, recent studies have found that DD does occur in the female population, but with reduced prevalence. The male-to-female ratio of DD varies between 7:1 and 15:1,[41] with a mean of about 5.9:1,[34] but in later life the prevalence in women increases to the same as in men.[3] Some investigators suggest that the disease symptoms are milder in women, and therefore may be systematically under-reported[17] Women are older at the time of their first operation, and have a higher recurrence rate[34] compared with men.[42,43] Several studies have also suggested a significantly stronger genetic element of DD in women. Two observations have supported this idea:

1. Familial cases of the disease predominantly in women.[40]
2. Higher sibling recurrence risk of DD in women compared with men.[34,44–46]

Table 1
Studies supporting environmental risk factors in Dupuytren disease

Study	Results That Support Environmental Risk Factors in DD
Finsen et al,[33] 2002	Family members were more likely to develop DD if they were residing in the same geographic area as their diseased relative
Srivastava et al,[30] 1989	The report of 10 cases of DD in patients from the Indian subcontinent who lived in the United Kingdom for several years before developing DD
Mandalia and Lowdon,[72] 2003; Beleta and Fores,[54] 2012	The report of DD present in only 1 identical twin may be the result of sole environmental factors such as rock climbing, or the disease may have developed at a later date in the other sibling
Zaworski and Mann,[19] 1979	A sporadic case in an African American with no evidence of familial clustering or interracial marital relationships. However, the patient had epilepsy and worked as a manual laborer
Furnas,[22] 1979; Richard-Kadio et al,[23] 1990; Mennen,[24] 1986; Aladin and Oni,[25] 2001; Maes,[26] 1979; Pai and Tseng,[27] 1994	These cases were sporadic with no family history of DD. There was a history of manual trauma in the male patients and a history of epilepsy in the female patients
Srivastava et al,[30] 1989	10 male cases (age range, 45–68 y) originating from the Indian subcontinent. None of the cases had a positive family history, but 8 out of 10 had a history of repetitive hand trauma
Lyall,[73] 1993; Beleta and Fores,[54] 2012	A twin study has shown that environmental factors are involved in disease pathogenesis because only 1 twin was affected with DD

Box 1
Risk factors associated with Dupuytren disease

Age

Gender

History of manual labor

Hand injury

History of smoking

Alcohol consumption

Epilepsy and antiepileptic medication

Diabetes mellitus (insulin dependent and non–insulin dependent)

Rock climbing

Carpal tunnel syndrome

Frozen shoulder

Rheumatoid arthritis

Hypercholesterolemia

Liver disease

Human immunodeficiency virus infection

Occupation, Trauma, Rock Climbing, Frozen Shoulder, Carpal Tunnel Syndrome, and Dupuytren Disease

On December 5, 1831, Baron Guillaume Dupuytren clearly identified the lesion of DD. In his lecture, Baron Dupuytren associated the disease with chronic local trauma caused by occupation. Several studies have supported the role of occupation as a causal factor in the pathogenesis of DD. However, around a year after Dupuytren's lecture, Goyrand contested the role of manual work and cited the case of his hospital manager with bilateral disease who had "never put the day of hard work"[5] and thus began the debate. Hand trauma, a history of manual labor,[47] hand injury, hand infection, elective hand surgery, or vibration exposure have been suggested as precipitating factors for DD.[47–49]

A recent study has concluded that patients with a history of frozen shoulder are 8 times more likely to develop DD.[50] Similarly, a history of carpal tunnel syndrome has been observed to be associated with an increased prevalence of DD.[51]

A further study has concluded that occupational history and social class have no bearing on DD development or progression. Early[8] in 1962 concluded that there was no significant difference in the prevalence of DD in manual and nonmanual workers. Contrary to these findings, Gudmundsson and colleagues[4] concluded a significant association between manual work and DD. Dasgupta

and Harrison[52] and Descatha and colleagues[53] found a positive correlation between vibration white finger and DD, and a more recent study to determine whether DD is more prevalent following repetitive trauma found that rock climbing increases the risk of disease development.[54]

Alcohol Consumption, Liver Disease, and Dupuytren Disease

Alcohol consumption and its association with DD is controversial. Several studies have found that alcohol consumption might be related to DD, whereas no significant relationship could be found in others. Two theories have been proposed for the correlation between DD and alcohol consumption:

- Alcohol consumption has been increasing over time, and this has been linked to increasing prevalence of DD.[6,55]
- The increasing reported prevalence of DD might be caused by increased recognition by health professionals and patients.

This possibility raises doubts on the direct impact that alcohol may have on DD. However, it should be noted that it is not alcohol consumption, per se, that seems to be a contributory factor for DD but rather the abuse of alcohol intake, especially over an extended time. In relation to this associated risk, liver disease has been found to be associated with DD as a separate associated factor.[56] Results of these studies need to be interpreted with caution. The results by Noble and colleagues[56] were in a cohort of patients with liver disease, and those by Lanting and colleagues[6] in a population aged more than 50 years, whereas it is already known that the prevalence of DD increases with age.[34]

Smoking and Dupuytren Disease

Some studies have shown a correlation between smoking habits and DD,[10,57,58] whereas others have shown none.[34] Because the prevalence of smoking is decreasing,[57] it is unlikely that increased risk is associated with smoking habits. In spite of this, cigarette smoking and increased alcohol consumption are more likely to result in surgical, rather than conservative, management of DD.[57] The opposite might be expected: that surgical management and risk of complications is higher in smokers and thus there would be a reduced rate of operative intervention; this study's response is that smokers tend to have greater severity of disease. However, smoking is not a diathesis factor (discussed later).

Hypercholesterolemia/Hypertriglyceridemia and Dupuytren Disease

A positive correlation has been found between DD and secondary hypercholesterolemia. It is also known that patients with DD are more likely to have increased serum triglyceride concentrations.[59,60] With an aging population, both hypercholesterolemia and DD are likely to become more prevalent, so this association may just be coincidence rather than cause and effect.

Diabetes Mellitus and Dupuytren Disease

The prevalence of diabetes mellitus is increasing.[61] Diabetes mellitus has been related to DD in numerous reports[56,61] and no associations have been found in others. Whether or not diabetes is an causal factor for DD, or whether the two conditions merely have a tendency to occur together, is debatable. Because most patients with diabetes mellitus do not get DD, it is unlikely that diabetes mellitus has an important role in the pathogenesis of DD. However, some patients presenting with DD have brought to light an underlying diagnosis of diabetes, and, as a result, surgeons and anesthetists should therefore be vigilant for diabetes when treating patients with DD.

Epilepsy/Epilepsy Medication and Dupuytren Disease

DD has been associated with epilepsy.[12] However, it is a fairly new association that almost parallels the introduction of phenobarbital and phenytoin. DD was not common in epileptics before the widespread use of these medicines but is very common in patients on long-term treatment with them. In some cases, the severity of DD seems to worsen following long-term treatment with phenobarbital. It is now thought that DD may be associated with these medical treatments for epilepsy rather than epilepsy itself.

Several hypotheses have been put forward regarding the possible effect of these drugs on the pathophysiology of DD. For instance, it is thought that the medication could be activating some genes, cytokine pathways, or increases in the level of growth factors. Other theories suggest that the liver might be involved given the high levels of aspartate transaminase (aspartate aminotransferase) and alanine transaminase (alanine aminotransferase) that have been detected in some studies. Moreover, epileptics have a higher incidence of Ledderhose disease and knuckle pads, which suggests a propensity to develop fibrotic diseases.

Human Immunodeficiency Virus and Dupuytren Disease

DD has been found to occur in around 6% to 36% of patients with human immunodeficiency virus (HIV).[62,63] The wide variation in prevalence of DD in patients infected with HIV may not be secondary to HIV infection but secondary to other causal factors. The association of HIV and DD requires further independent validation.

Rheumatoid Arthritis and Dupuytren Disease

Rheumatoid arthritis is the only condition so far noted to be negatively associated with DD. A cross-sectional study from Manchester, United Kingdom, performed in 1984, examined the hands of 392 patients with rheumatoid arthritis.[64] There was a significantly reduced prevalence rate of DD in patients with a diagnosis of rheumatoid arthritis, suggesting a genetic protective factor against the disease.[64]

In summary, there are conflicting data about many of the environmental associations thought to be important in DD, which implies that most of these factors do not exert a strong influence on the prevalence of the disease.

However, some environmental factors have reliably been associated with postsurgical recurrence and/or spread of DD, including male gender and a young age of onset; these form part of the so-called Dupuytren diathesis.

DUPUYTREN DIATHESIS: A PREDICTOR FOR DISEASE RECURRENCE

Diathesis describes a condition, constitution, or morbid habit that predisposes an individual to a particular disease. The DD diathesis is a term first coined by Hueston,[65] relating to certain characteristics of the disease and dictating an aggressive course and greater tendency for recurrence after surgical treatment. Hueston[65] described 4 factors as part of the DD diathesis: bilateral disease (described as bilateral palmar lesions), family history of DD, ectopic lesions (DD found outside the palmar surface), and ethnicity.[65,66] Hueston's[65] study on the DD diathesis distinguished between patients who developed recurrence and extension, with recurrence occurring more frequently.

The degree of diathesis is considered highly significant in predicting recurrence and extension of DD following surgical management. Recurrence of DD is problematic for the patient and the surgeon, because repeat surgery conveys additional risk of complications. Prognostic indicators of risks associated with surgery are important, therefore, for shared decision-making with the patient.[67]

Recurrence rates reported following fasciectomy range between 12% and 73%.[68] Recurrence refers to the development of disease at the same location and can be divided into 2 types:

1. True recurrence: development of new DD tissue within the area of previous surgery and false recurrence.
2. False recurrence: development of scar and joint contracture not directly related to DD.

Extension describes the development of disease away from the area of surgery.[68]

Hueston's[65] original definition was updated to include young age at onset (<50 years of age) and male gender.[67] This study, which revisited the original diathesis, did not include ethnicity, because all patients in the study cohort were white.[67] **Table 2** summarizes the original and new diathesis for DD.

The presence of all 5 new DD diathesis factors in a patient increases the risk of recurrent DD by 71% compared with a baseline risk of 23% in those patients with DD with only 1 of the new DD diathesis factors.[67]

One of the most significant common factors in relation to disease recurrence, and part of the DD diathesis, is a positive family history.[34] It was first recognized that DD might have some genetic predisposition even before DNA and genes were discovered.[8] Although many of the environmental factors mentioned earlier have only weak or controversial evidence behind them, evidence for the genetic aspects of DD have steadily gained over the years.[44]

Several studies on the genetic origin of DD have been performed.[17,31,34,69–71] Studies have examined the mode of inheritance and also potential genetic pathways to elucidate the heritable cause of DD. Multiple reports describe DD as an autosomal dominant disease with varying penetrance (estimated level of penetrance is 18%).[32,40] A review of the inheritance pattern of DD in 1999 suggested that recessive inheritance still remains a viable hypothesis for DD.[17] Nevertheless, most of the reports still tend to favor an autosomal dominant mode with variable penetrance[34] (provided the disease is monogenic). Of note, many published studies point toward DD being a polygenic disease, given the large numbers of genes that have been found to be involved in the disease.[31,32,70,71]

The genetics of DD is extensive and there is a clear translation from the clinical assessment of patients with a DD diathesis to the scientific data being analyzed now and into the future.

REFERENCES

1. Elliot D. The early history of contracture of the palmar fascia. Part 1: the origin of the disease: the curse of the MacCrimmons: the hand of benediction: cline's contracture. J Hand Surg Br 1988; 13(3):246–53.
2. Shih B, Bayat A. Scientific understanding and clinical management of Dupuytren disease. Nat Rev Rheumatol 2010;6:715–26.
3. Ross DC. Epidemiology of Dupuytren's disease. Hand Clin 1999;15(1):53–62.
4. Gudmundsson KG, Arngrimsson R, Sigfusson N, et al. Epidemiology of Dupuytren's disease: clinical, serological, and social assessment. The Reykjavik Study. J Clin Epidemiol 2000;53(3):291–6.
5. Thurston AJ. Dupuytren's disease. J Bone Joint Surg Br 2003;85:469–77.
6. Lanting R, van den Heuvel ER, Westerink B, et al. Prevalence of Dupuytren disease in the Netherlands. Plast Reconstr Surg 2013;132(2):394–403.
7. Bayat A, McGrouther DA. Management of Dupuytren's disease—clear advice for an elusive condition. Ann R Coll Surg Engl 2006;88(1):3–8.
8. Early PF. Population studies in Dupuytren's contracture. J Bone Joint Surg Br 1962;44:602–13.
9. Mikkelsen OA. The prevalence of Dupuytren's disease in Norway. A study in a representative population sample of the municipality of Haugesund. Acta Chir Scand 1972;138(7):695–700.
10. Gudmundsson KG, Arngrimsson R, Jonsson T. Prevalence of joint complaints amongst individuals with Dupuytren's disease-from the Reykjavik study. Scand J Rheumatol 1999;28(5):300–4.
11. Quintana Guitian A. Various epidemiologic aspects of Dupuytren's disease. Ann Chir Main 1988;7:256–62.
12. Skoog T. Dupuytren's contracture with special reference to aetiology and improved surgical treatment,

Table 2 Original and new diathesis for Dupuytren disease	
Original DD Diathesis Factors	**New DD Diathesis Factors**
Bilateral DD	Bilateral disease
Family history of DD	Family history of DD
Ectopic disease (nonspecific)	Ectopic disease (specific to Garrod pads)
Ethnicity	Young age at onset (<50 y of age)
—	Male gender
—	Ethnicity

its occurrence in epileptics, note on knuckle pads. Acta Chir Scand Suppl 1948;96(39):25–175.

13. Brenner P, Krause-Bergmann A, Van VH. Die Dupuytren- Kontraktur in Norddeutschland. Epidemiologische Erfassungsstudie anhand von 500 Fällen. Unfallchirurg 2001;104:303–11 [in German].

14. Hindocha S, McGrouther DA, Bayat A. Epidemiological evaluation of Dupuytren's disease incidence and prevalence rates in relation to etiology. Hand (N Y) 2009;4:256–69.

15. Zerajic D, Finsen V. Dupuytren's disease in Bosnia and Herzegovina. An epidemiological study. BMC Musculoskelet Disord 2002;29(5):10.

16. McFarlane RM. On the origin and spread of Dupuytren's disease. J Hand Surg Am 2002;27:385–90.

17. Burge P. Genetics of Dupuytren's disease. Hand Clin 1999;15(1):63–71.

18. Plasse JS. Dupuytren's contracture in a black patient. Plast Reconstr Surg 1979;64(2):250.

19. Zaworski RE, Mann RJ. Dupuytren's contracture in a black patient. Plast Reconstr Surg 1979;63(1): 122–4.

20. Sladicka MS, Benfanti P, Raab M, et al. Dupuytren's contracture in the black population: a case report and review of the literature. J Hand Surg Am 1996; 21(5):898–9.

21. Swartz WM, Lalonde DH. MOD-PS(SM) CME article: Dupuytren's disease. Plast Reconstr Surg 2008; 121(4 Suppl):1–10.

22. Furnas DW. Dupuytren's contracture in a black patient in East Africa. Plast Reconstr Surg 1979; 64(2):250–1.

23. Richard-Kadio M, Guedegbe F, Dick R, et al. Dupuytren's contracture: review of the literature. Case report of a black African. Med Trop (Mars) 1990; 50(3):311–3 [in French].

24. Mennen U. Dupuytren's contracture in the Negro. J Hand Surg Br 1986;11(1):61–4.

25. Aladin A, Oni JA. Bilateral Dupuytren's contracture in a black patient. Int J Clin Pract 2001;55(9):641–2.

26. Maes J. Dupuytren's contracture in an oriental patient. Plast Reconstr Surg 1979;64(2):251.

27. Pai CH, Tseng CH. Dupuytren's contracture: report of a Taiwanese case. J Formos Med Assoc 1994; 93(8):724–6.

28. Liu YIH, Chen WY. Dupuytren's disease among the Chinese in Taiwan. J Hand Surg Am 1991;16(5): 779–86.

29. Vathana P, Setpakdi A, Srimongkol T. Dupuytren's contracture in Thailand. Bull Hosp Jt Dis Orthop Inst 1990;50(1):41–7.

30. Srivastava S, Nancarrow J, Cort DF. Dupuytren's disease in patients from the Indian sub-continent. Report of ten cases. J Hand Surg Br 1989;14(1): 32–4.

31. Hu FZ, Nystrom A, Ahmed A, et al. Mapping of an autosomal dominant gene for Dupuytren's contracture to chromosome 16q in a Swedish family. Clin Genet 2005;68(5):424–9.

32. Ling RS. The genetic factor in Dupuytren's disease. J Bone Joint Surg 1963;45:709–18.

33. Finsen V, Dalen H, Nesheim J. The prevalence of Dupuytren's disease among different ethnic groups in northern Norway. J Hand Surg Am 2002;27(1):115–7.

34. Hindocha S, John S, Stanley JK, et al. The heritability of Dupuytren's disease: familial aggregation and its clinical significance. J Hand Surg Am 2006;31: 204–10.

35. Paller AS, Hebert AA. Knuckle pads in children. JAMA 1986;141:915.

36. Rao GS, Luthra PK. Dupuytren's disease of the foot in children; a report of three cases. Br J Plast Surg 1988;41(3):313–5.

37. Rhomberg M, Rainer C, Gardetto A, et al. Dupuytren's disease in children–differential diagnosis. J Pediatr Surg 2002;37(4):E7.

38. Lane JG, Hankin FM. Dupuytren's contracture in an adolescent. Am Fam Physician 1988;37(4):133–6.

39. Bebbington A, Savage R. Dupuytren's disease in an infant. J Bone Joint Surg Br 2005;87:111–3.

40. Matthews P. Familial Dupuytren's contracture with predominantly female expression. Br J Plast Surg 1979;32(2):120–3.

41. Gudmundsson KG, Arngrimsson R, Sigfusson N, et al. Increased total mortality and cancer mortality in men with Dupuytren's disease. A 15 year follow-up study. J Clin Epidemiol 2002;55(1):5–10.

42. Wilbrand S, Ekbom A, Gerdin B. The sex ratio and rate of reoperation for Dupuytren's contracture in men and women. J Hand Surg Br 1999;24:456–9.

43. Wurster-Hill DH, Brown F, Park JP, et al. Cytogenetic studies in Dupuytren contracture. Am J Hum Genet 1988;43(3):285–92.

44. Capstic R, Bragg T, Giele H, et al. Sibling recurrence risk in Dupuytren's disease. J Hand Surg 2012;38(4): 424–9.

45. Casalone R, Mazzola D, Meroni E, et al. Cytogenetic and interphase cytogenetic analyses reveal chromosome instability but no clonal trisomy 8 in Dupuytren contracture. Cancer Genet Cytogenet 1997;99(1): 73–6.

46. Dal Cin P, De Smet L, Sciot R, et al. Trisomy 7 and trisomy 8 in dividing and non dividing tumour cells in Dupuytren's disease. Cancer Genet Cytogenet 1999;108(2):137–40.

47. De la Caffiniere JY, Wagner R, Etscheid J, et al. Manual labor and Dupuytren disease. The results of a computerized survey in the field of iron metallurgy. Ann Chir Main 1983;2(1):66–72.

48. Luck JV. Dupuytren's contracture: a new concept of the pathogenesis correlated with surgical management. J Bone Joint Surg Am 1959;41:635.

49. McFarlane RM. Dupuytren's disease: relation to work injury. J Hand Surg Am 1991;16(5):775–9.

50. Smith SP, Devaraj VS, Bunker TD. The association between frozen shoulder and Dupuytren's disease. J Shoulder Elbow Surg 2001;10(2):149–51.

51. Bonnici AV, Birjandi F, Spencer JD, et al. Chromosomal abnormalities in Dupuytren's contracture and carpal tunnel syndrome. J Hand Surg Br 1992; 17(3):349–55.

52. Dasgupta AK, Harrison J. Effects of vibration on the hand-arm system of miners in India. Occup Med (Lond) 1996;46:71.

53. Descatha A, Bodin J, Ha C, et al. Heavy manual work, exposure to vibration and Dupuytren's disease? Results of a surveillance program for musculoskeletal disorders. Occup Environ Med 2012; 69(4):296–9.

54. Beleta H, Fores J. Dupuytren's disease in a rock climber with an unaffected identical twin. J Hand Surg Eur 2012;39(3):313–4.

55. Arafa M, Noble J, Royle SG, et al. Dupuytren's and epilepsy revisited. J Hand Surg Br 1992;17(2): 221–4.

56. Noble J, Heathcote JG, Cohen H. Diabetes mellitus in the aetiology of Dupuytren's disease. J Bone Joint Surg Br 1984;66:322–5.

57. Burge P, Hoy G, Regan P, et al. Smoking, alcohol and the risk of Dupuytren's contracture. J Bone Joint Surg Br 1997;79:206–10.

58. Weinstein AL, Haddock NT, Sharma S. Dupuytren's disease in the Hispanic population: a 10 year retrospective review. Plast Reconstr Surg 2011;128(6): 1251–6.

59. Sanderson PL, Morris MA, Stanley JK, et al. Lipids and Dupuytren's disease. J Bone Joint Surg Br 1992;74:923–7.

60. Sergovich FR, Botz JS, McFarlane RM. Nonrandom cytogenetic abnormalities in Dupuytren's disease. N Engl J Med 1983;308(3):162–3.

61. Arkkila PE, Kantola IM, Vilkari JS. Dupuytren's disease: association with chronic diabetic complications. J Rheumatol 1997;24(1):153–9.

62. Bower M, Nelson M, Gazzard BG. Dupuytren's contractures in patients infected with HIV. BMJ 1990; 300(6718):164–5.

63. French PD, Kitchen VS, Harris JR. Prevalence of Dupuytren's contracture in patients infected with HIV. BMJ 1990;301(6758):967.

64. Arafa M, Steingold RF, Noble J. The incidence of Dupuytren's disease in patients with rheumatoid arthritis. J Hand Surg Br 1984;9(2):165–6.

65. Hueston JT. The Dupuytren's diathesis. London: Churchill Livingstone; 1963. p. 51–63.

66. Kaur S, Forsman M, Ryhänen J, et al. No gene copy number changes in Dupuytren's contracture by array comparative genomic hybridization. Cancer Genet Cytogenet 2008;183(1):6–8.

67. Hindocha S, Stanley JK, Watson S, et al. Dupuytren's diathesis revisited: evaluation of prognostic indicators for risk of disease recurrence. J Hand Surg Am 2006;31(10):1626–34.

68. Werker PM, Pess GM, van Rijssen AL, et al. Correction of contracture and recurrence rates of Dupuytren contracture following invasive treatment: the importance of clear definitions. J Hand Surg Am 2012;37(10):2095–105.e7.

69. Badalamente MA, Sampson SP, Hurst LC, et al. The role of transforming growth factor beta in Dupuytren's disease. J Hand Surg Am 1996; 21(2):210–5.

70. Bayat A, Watson S, Stanley JK, et al. Genetic susceptibility to Dupuytren's disease: association of Zf9 transcription factor gene. Plast Reconstr Surg 2002;111(7):2133–9.

71. Lee LC, Zhang AY, Chong AK, et al. Expression of a novel gene, MafB, in Dupuytren's disease. J Hand Surg Am 2006;31(2):211–8.

72. Mandalia VI, Lowdon MR. Dupuytren's disease in a child: a case report. J Pediatr Orthop B 2003; 12(3):198–9.

73. Lyall HA. Dupuytren's disease in identical twins. J Hand Surg 1993;18(3):368.

Normal and Pathologic Anatomy of Dupuytren Disease

Stephen J. Leibovic, MD, MS[a,b,*]

KEYWORDS

- Normal anatomy • Pathologic anatomy • Dupuytren disease • Treatment

KEY POINTS

- Knowledge of the normal fascial anatomy of the hand is essential to understand the pathologic anatomy of Dupuytren disease. Understanding the pathologic anatomy is, in turn, essential for safe treatment of the condition.
- Nodules occur in somewhat unpredictable locations, usually in the layer of tissue between the superficial palmar fascia and the skin.
- Cords occur in predictable locations, forming along the course of normal fascial bands, changing their direction and relationships to other structures as they thicken and contract.
- Disparate and conflicting terminology can be reconciled into a uniform nomenclature for describing the fascial bands and diseased cords of Dupuytren contracture.

INTRODUCTION

Safe treatment of Dupuytren disease, whether by collagenase injection, needle aponeurotomy, or surgery, relies on a thorough understanding of the pertinent normal and pathologic anatomy. Elements of diseased fascia occur in predictable locations throughout the hand, and knowledge of their locations is based on an understanding of the normal anatomy that precedes the formation of abnormal cords. Terminology referring to both normal and diseased Dupuytren anatomy has become more uniform but still lacks consistency among authors and anatomists. This article describes the current state of knowledge of the relevant anatomy and reconciles some disparities in nomenclature. To avoid confusion in nomenclature the author uses a uniform naming paradigm. Other terms that have been used to name the same anatomic structures are cross referenced in **Table 1**.

PATHOGENESIS

Dupuytren disease occurs in 2 primary forms: nodules and cords. Nodules precede cords and go through 3 stages of development: The (first) proliferative stage, the (second) involutional stage, and the (third) residual stage.[1] It is during this evolution that cords appear. In the proliferative phase, nodules are filled with myofibroblasts in a dense, chaotic organization. They are most often found in areas of the hand rich in fat, usually attached to the skin or the superficial palmar fascia, or occurring in the space between them. Vessels in the nodule appear histologically to have thicker walls than normal palmar vessels, and demonstrate some occlusion of their lumens,[2] leading Murrell to postulate that localized ischemia is involved in the pathogenesis of nodules and cords. Various factors, including cytokines, transforming growth factor (TGF)-β1, and free radicals are produced in and around the nodules and cords

[a] Department of Orthopedic Surgery and Division of Plastic and Reconstructive Surgery, Virginia Commonwealth University, Richmond, VA 23298, USA; [b] Virginia Hand Center, 2819 N. Parham Road, Suite 100, Richmond, VA 23294, USA
* Virginia Hand Center, 2819 N. Parham Road, Suite 100, Richmond, VA 23294.
E-mail address: steve@leibovic.org

Hand Clin 34 (2018) 315–329
https://doi.org/10.1016/j.hcl.2018.04.001

Table 1
Reconciliation of Dupuytren terminology

Terminology Used in This Article	Alternate and Equivalent Terminology
Palmar aponeurosis	Superficial palmar fascia Central aponeurosis
Natatory ligament	Superficial transverse ligament (McGrouther); (superficial transverse) interdigital ligament (Gosset)
Natatory ligament (extension to thumb)	Distal commissural ligament
Superficial transverse palmar ligament	Deep transverse fibers (McGrouther) Transverse ligament of the palmar aponeurosis
Superficial transverse palmar ligament (extension to the thumb)	Proximal commissural ligament
Septae of Legueu and Juvara	None
Deep transverse metacarpal ligament	Deep transverse metacarpal fibers (McGrouther) Deep aponeurosis (Gosset)
Pretendinous bands	Longitudinal fibers to skin (McGrouther)
Bifurcated pretendinous band/spiral band, with insertion into metacarpophalangeal capsule and P1 via web space coalescence to lateral digital sheet	Longitudinal fibers to finger (McGrouther)
Bifurcated pretendinous band/spiral band, with insertion to tendon sheath via web space coalescence	Longitudinal fibers to tendon sheath (McGrouther)
Vertical fibers	Grapow vertical bands
Isolated digital cord	Unnamed cord involving only lateral digital sheet (Gosset) Ulnar spiral cord of small finger (Hueston, McFarlane)
Spiral band	Deep extension (of pretendinous band) (Gosset) Oblique band (Hettiaratchy)

leading to an increased production of type III collagen, which begins to appear and mature in the second, involutional or contractile phase of the nodule. TGF-β1 promotes fibroblast differentiation into myofibroblasts, which precipitates cord contraction. In addition, fibroblast growth factor, platelet-derived growth factor, and TGF-α are more commonly found in Dupuytren tissue.[3] As the disease progresses, the collagen matures, forming more well-defined cords. The myofibroblasts continue to contract and "pucker" the nascent collagen cords.[4] Collagenase is present in diseased Dupuytren tissue, which breaks down the "puckered" cords, allowing them to re-form cross links in an ever more shortened position as the myofibroblasts contract, leading to progressive contracture. Finally, in the third, residual stage of nodule formation, there is established contracture mediated by the cords, and the nodules appear hypocellular; those cells that remain appear aged and hypoactive. Active myofibroblasts are scarce. Therefore, during the evolution of Dupuytren contracture, both the number and the activity of myofibroblasts varies according to the phase of development.

But where do the cords occur? Some believe[5] that nodules and cords arise de novo in regions in which there are no normal fascial structures, the so-called extrinsic theory. It is now generally accepted, however, that cords mostly arise from normal fascial structures (the intrinsic theory) and present as thickened diseased fascia.[6-9] So, whereas the nodules appear in random locations between the superficial palmar fascia and the skin, cords arise in largely predictable loci. This lends credence to Gosset's[10] belief that cords and nodules are separate forms of the disease that originate in different tissues. Gosset[10] states "the relations (of cords) to the neurovascular elements are classical and anatomically predictable." They occur as thickenings of existing normal fascial bands and combinations of bands. Hence an understanding of the normal fascial anatomy of the hand is required to understand and safely address the thickened cords.

NORMAL ANATOMY OF THE PALMAR FASCIA

Palmar and digital fascia forms an important stabilizing structure in the hand that imparts a degree of firmness of the glabrous skin of the palm and fingers and protection of the underlying anatomic structures. Absence of fascial components imparts a degree of flexibility to the dorsal skin. Separated by anatomists into named structures, the fascia forms a complex and interconnected system throughout the hand. In many locations, different named structures blend and coalesce in a manner that defies anatomic separation. The surgeon must not expect to be always able to

separate these structures from each other in either the normal or the diseased state, but rather must understand how they blend together and coalesce.

The palmar aponeurosis is roughly triangular in shape, lying in a coronal plane deep to the skin (**Fig. 1**). Its origin is at the wrist in close proximity to the palmaris longus when that tendon exists. As it diverges from the wrist, it splits into longitudinal strips, or pretendinous bands, coursing toward the fingers. In a sagittal plane, the fibers divide into 3 groups (**Fig. 2**). The most superficial fibers of the pretendinous bands course toward the skin where they attach, mostly between the distal palmar crease and the proximal digital crease, in what McGrouther[11] termed longitudinal fibers to the skin and McFarlane[7] termed pretendinous bands, with fascial insertion to skin (see

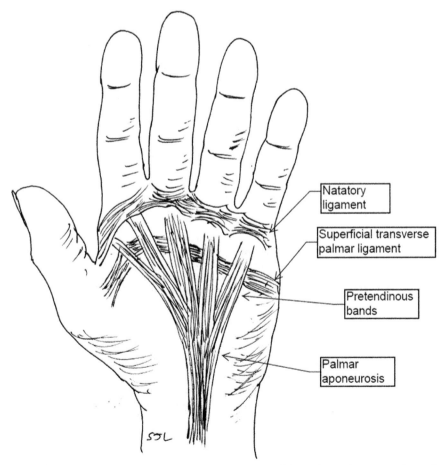

Fig. 1. The palmar aponeurosis has its origin near the termination of the palmaris longus tendon, when it is present. It lies in the coronal plane. It divides into a pretendinous band coursing to each of the fingers (and sometimes the thumb). The pretendinous bands continue distally as the spiral bands (see **Fig. 11**). Lying deep to the pretendinous bands, the superficial transverse palmar ligament is mostly in the coronal plane. At the web spaces, the natatory ligament has a more 3-dimensional deep configuration than the superficial transverse palmar ligament; only the most superficial layer of the natatory ligament is shown here. (*Courtesy of* S. Leibovic, MD, Richmond, VA.)

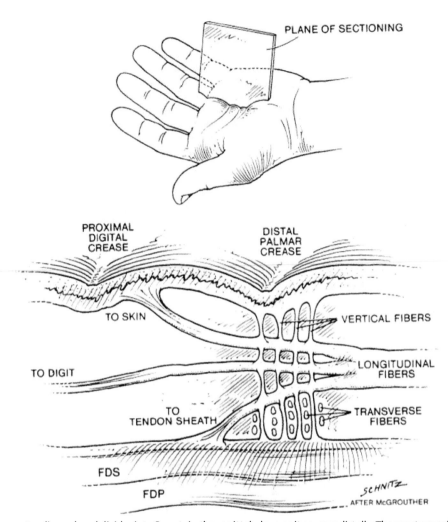

Fig. 2. The pretendinous band divides into 3 parts in the sagittal plane as it courses distally. The most superficial fibers insert into the skin. The intermediate part continues as the spiral band and rotates (twists) 90° as it courses toward the web space coalescence and on to the lateral digital sheet. The deepest part inserts into the MP joint capsule and the flexor tendon sheath. FDS, flexor digitorum superficialis; FDP, flexor digitorum profundus. (*From* Strickland JW, Leibovic SJ. Anatomy and pathogenesis of the digital cords and nodules. Hand Clin 1991;7(4):645–57; with permission.)

Table 1). Intermediate-depth fibers from the pretendinous bands bifurcate into 2 separate strips, which diverge around the metacarpal head and rotate (twist) 90° to come to lie in the sagittal plane (**Fig. 3**). From the point of their bifurcation, these fibers are no longer called pretendinous bands but rather the spiral band or the deep extension of the pretendinous band. Each spiral band hugs the metacarpophalangeal (MP) joint capsule as it diverges from the palm, then rotates 90° as the bandlike structure continues into the web space (**Figs. 3** and **4**). Most of these fibers coalesce in the web space in a conjoined mass of fascia termed the web space coalescence by Leibovic.[9] Distal to the web space coalescence they continue out in the finger on each side,

forming the lateral digital sheet (**Fig. 5**). The deepest fibers from the pretendinous bands course distally as they dive deeper both proximal and distal to the transverse fibers of the palmar aponeurosis (see **Fig. 2**) in what McGrouther has further subdivided into the deepest 3(b) layer and a somewhat more superficial 3(a) layer.[11] These deep fibers attach to the MP joint capsule and the flexor tendon sheath.

Running perpendicular to the pretendinous bands, all in the coronal plane, are 2 sets of transverse fibers in the palm (see **Figs. 3** and **4**). The first, the superficial transverse palmar ligament, lies at the level of the distal palmar crease. At its ulnar-most border it attaches to the skin and the hypothenar fascia, which itself is continuous

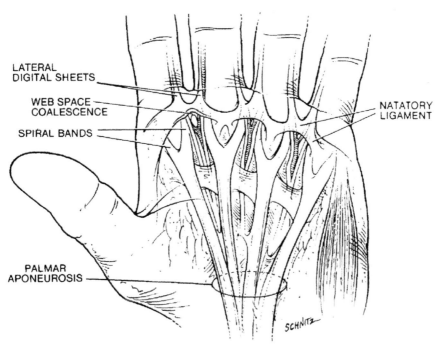

LATERAL
DIGITAL SHEETS

WEB SPACE
COALESCENCE

SPIRAL BANDS

NATATORY
LIGAMENT

PALMAR
APONEUROSIS

SCHNITz

Fig. 3. As the pretendinous bands divide into 2, they become the spiral bands that rotate (twist) 90° as they course around the metacarpal head to insert into the web space coalescence. Here, they are under the most superficial portions of the natatory ligament, which itself sends deep fibers into the web space coalescence. The neurovascular bundle is lateral to the pretendinous band but medial to the lateral digital sheet. The web space coalescence is deep to the neurovascular bundle. (*From* Strickland JW, Leibovic SJ. Anatomy and pathogenesis of the digital cords and nodules. Hand Clin 1991;7(4):645–57; with permission.)

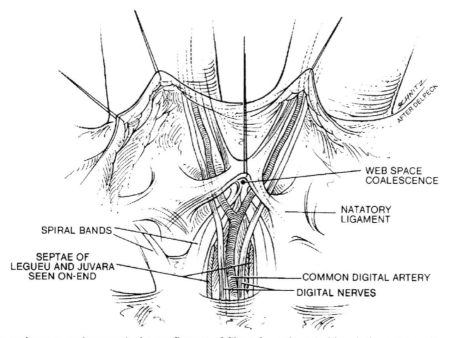

SCHNITz
AFTER DELPECK

WEB SPACE
COALESCENCE

NATATORY
LIGAMENT

SPIRAL BANDS

SEPTAE OF
LEGUEU AND JUVARA
SEEN ON-END

COMMON DIGITAL ARTERY

DIGITAL NERVES

Fig. 4. The web space coalescence is the confluence of fibers from the spiral band, the natatory ligament, the septae of Legueu and Juvara, and the lateral digital sheet. Note here the 3-dimensional configuration of the natatory ligament. Particularly in fascia diseased with Dupuytren contracture, it is usually not possible to separate out all the component anatomic contributions. (*From* Strickland JW, Leibovic SJ. Anatomy and pathogenesis of the digital cords and nodules. Hand Clin 1991;7(4):645–57; with permission.)

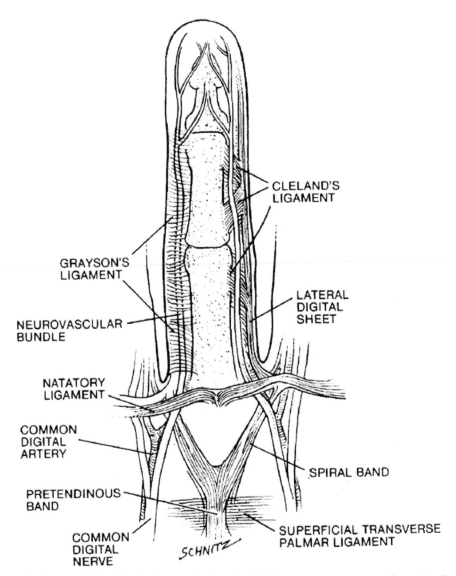

Fig. 5. Normal palmar and digital fascia that may be involved in Dupuytren contracture. The pretendinous band divides into the 2 spiral bands that course to the web space coalescence. The natatory ligament and the lateral digital sheet also contribute to the web space coalescence. The Cleland ligaments extend from the lateral digital sheet dorsally in the finger, whereas Grayson ligaments extend from the lateral digital sheet in a volar direction in the finger toward the flexor sheath and the periosteum. (*From* Strickland JW, Leibovic SJ. Anatomy and pathogenesis of the digital cords and nodules. Hand Clin 1991;7(4):645–57; with permission.)

distally with Grayson ligaments and a slip of the abductor digiti quinti tendon.[12] At its radial-most border, the superficial transverse palmar ligament attaches to the thenar fascia. It lies mostly in the coronal plane, diverging somewhat out of that plane in the first web space. It courses deep to the pretendinous bands and is intimately connected to them at areas of intersection.

The second set of transverse fibers in the palm, the natatory ligament, lies at the level of, and courses between, all 4 web spaces. Unlike the superficial transverse palmar ligament, which lies mostly in the coronal plane, the natatory ligament is more 3-dimensional. Although its most superficial extent is just below the skin, it sends fibers deep to each side of the flexor tendon, attaching to the flexor sheath and the MP joint. In addition, it sends fibers deep toward, and becomes part of, the web space coalescence. Its location and morphology cause it to tighten with finger abduction and also with independent flexion of each MP joint.

Emanating from the deep surface of the palmar aponeurosis are the 8 septae of Legueu and Juvara. These course in the sagittal plane between the palmar aponeurosis and the interosseous muscle fascia, metacarpals, and the deep transverse metacarpal ligament (**Figs. 6–8**). Seven compartments are formed. Four contain the flexor tendons to all 4 fingers, and 3 contain the neurovascular bundles and lumbricals to the second, third, and fourth interspaces. The radial neurovascular bundle to the index finger and the ulnar neurovascular bundle to the small finger are without such compartments. In addition to providing protection to these structures, these septae anchor the overlying fascia, providing an additional proximal pulley for these flexor tendons, which provides added mechanical advantage in finger flexion.[13]

Grapow fibers course between the superficial palmar fascia and the dermis. They assist in anchoring the glabrous skin to the underlying structures in the palm.[13] They can thicken, which causes thickening of the skin ("pseudocallus"), often one of the earliest manifestations of Dupuytren disease. The septae of Legueu and Juvara and the vertical bands of Grapow are the only fibers associated with Dupuytren contracture that course primarily in the sagittal plane. Distally,

the septae of Legueu and Juvara also blend into the web space coalescence of Leibovic.

NORMAL ANATOMY OF THE DIGITAL FASCIA

As fibers from the web space coalescence of Leibovic course distally in the fingers they form a sheet of fibers in the sagittal plane, termed the lateral digital sheet (see **Fig. 2**; **Fig. 9**). It lies superficial to the extensor mechanism and extends toward the volar side of the digits as far as the Grayson ligaments. The lateral digital sheet provides protection for the neurovascular bundle as it courses distally in the digit. Fascial projections from the lateral digital sheet emerge sporadically in an inward radial direction and insert into the flexor sheath, joint capsule, and phalangeal periosteum. On the volar side, these projections are known as Grayson ligaments, whereas on the dorsal side they are known as Cleland ligaments. In between the septae formed by these projections is fat. Components of the lateral digital sheet lie volar to the axis of rotation of the proximal interphalangeal (PIP) joint.

If we follow the course of the pretendinous band distally (see **Fig. 5**), parts of it become the spiral band, which in turn forms part of the web space coalescence and finally, distal to the web space,

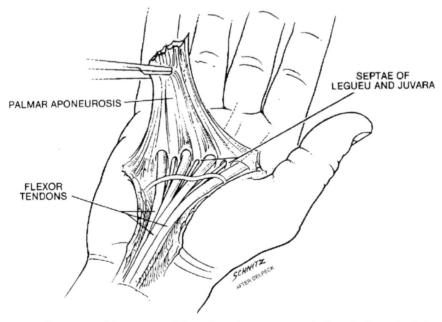

Fig. 6. The septae of Legueu and Juvara extend from the palmar aponeurosis deep, in the sagittal plane, and provide protection to the neurovascular bundles, flexor tendons, and intrinsic muscles that they surround. They contribute to the web space coalescence but are rarely involved in Dupuytren disease. (*From* Strickland JW, Leibovic SJ. Anatomy and pathogenesis of the digital cords and nodules. Hand Clin 1991;7(4):645–57; with permission.)

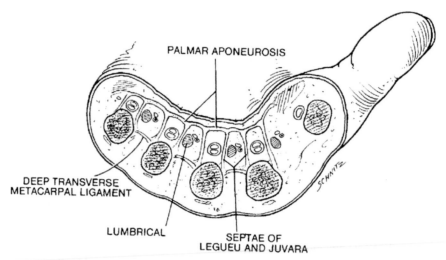

Fig. 7. The septae of Legueu and Juvara form 7 compartments, protecting the neurovascular bundles and flexor tendons. The border neurovascular bundles (radial for the index and ulnar for the small fingers) are unprotected by these septae. (*From* Strickland JW, Leibovic SJ. Anatomy and pathogenesis of the digital cords and nodules. Hand Clin 1991;7(4):645–57; with permission.)

this fascia merges with the lateral digital sheet. As the neurovascular bundle courses from distal to proximal, it begins lateral to the pretendinous band. The spiral band diverges to the lateral sides of the metacarpal and passes under the neurovascular bundle so that the web space coalescence, continuous with the spiral band, lies lateral to the neurovascular bundle. The lateral digital sheet, therefore, also lies lateral to the neurovascular bundle. The retrovascular band lies deep to the neurovascular bundle, extending beyond the distal interphalangeal joint (DIP). It originates from the periosteum of the proximal phalanx, and attaches to the lateral surface of the distal phalanx.[8]

PATHOLOGIC ANATOMY

Predictable pathologic features characterize patients with Dupuytren contracture. Perhaps as early as 15 BC, the characteristic flexion deformity

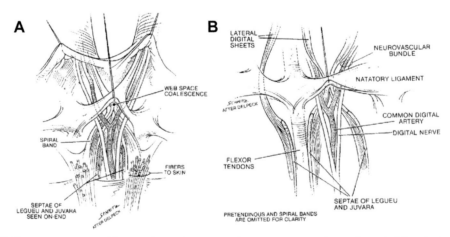

Fig. 8. (*A*) The components making up the web space coalescence are seen here: the spiral band, the septae of Legueu and Juvara, the natatory ligament, and the lateral digital sheet. The web space coalescence is seen beneath (deep to) the nerve and artery, which lie lateral to the proximal part of the spiral band and septae of Legueu and Juvara, but medial to the lateral digital sheet. (*B*) The septae of Legueu and Juvara lie in the sagittal plane and surround the flexor tendons, protecting them and the neurovascular bundles. (*From* Strickland JW, Leibovic SJ. Anatomy and pathogenesis of the digital cords and nodules. Hand Clin 1991;7(4):645–57; with permission.)

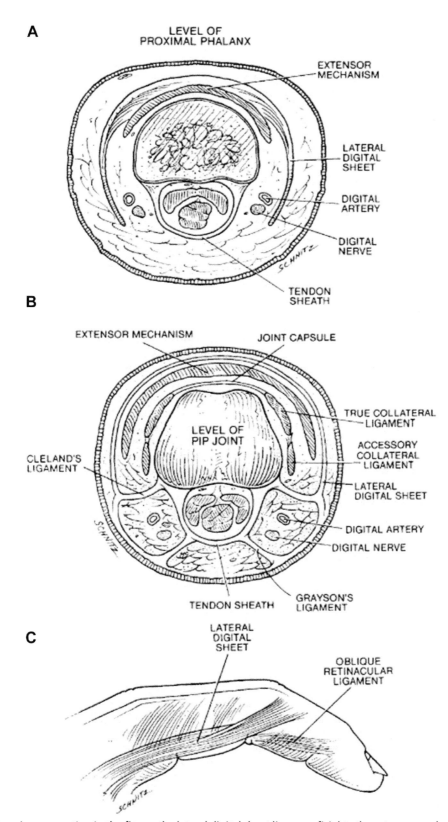

A LEVEL OF PROXIMAL PHALANX

EXTENSOR MECHANISM

LATERAL DIGITAL SHEET

DIGITAL ARTERY

DIGITAL NERVE

TENDON SHEATH

B

EXTENSOR MECHANISM   JOINT CAPSULE

LEVEL OF PIP JOINT

TRUE COLLATERAL LIGAMENT

ACCESSORY COLLATERAL LIGAMENT

LATERAL DIGITAL SHEET

DIGITAL ARTERY

DIGITAL NERVE

CLELAND'S LIGAMENT

TENDON SHEATH   GRAYSON'S LIGAMENT

C LATERAL DIGITAL SHEET

OBLIQUE RETINACULAR LIGAMENT

Fig. 9. Seen in cross section in the finger, the lateral digital sheet lies superficial to the extensor mechanism. It has components extending volar to both the PIP and the DIP joints, and its contraction can cause a flexion contracture of these joints. (*A*) Cross section through the proximal phalanx. (*B*) Cross section at the proximal interphalangeal joint. (*C*) Lateral view of finger. (*From* Strickland JW, Leibovic SJ. Anatomy and pathogenesis of the digital cords and nodules. Hand Clin 1991;7(4):645–57; with permission.)

of ring and small fingers was depicted in sculptures of Sabazius, a god of the Thracians and Phrygians who was depicted with humanlike physical traits.[14] Other colorful references, such as the "curse of the MacCrimmons," originated as members of a Scottish clan of bagpipers found themselves unable to play their instruments because of progressive digital contractures.

The disease often manifests first with nodules occurring between the skin and the superficial palmar fascia. Pits may occur as the most superficial fibers of the pretendinous band and the vertical bands of Grapow, inserting into the skin, begin to contract and draw the skin down.

Contracture most often begins with thickening of the pretendinous band into a pretendinous cord over the ring finger ray. The natatory ligaments may thicken and contract, which results in limitation of finger abduction and occasionally of finger flexion. Contracture of this confluence can cause PIP joint contractures as the web space coalescence and contiguous portions of the lateral digital sheet lie in a volar position with respect to the PIP joint. Surgical separation of the formerly contiguous but unaffected structures becomes more difficult as disease progressively infiltrates the fascial structures.

As disease infiltrates the palmar fascia, the confluence of the pretendinous band, spiral band, web space coalescence, and lateral digital sheet begins to thicken and contract. The normal anatomy, whereby the neurovascular bundle begins lateral (with respect to the midline of each finger) to the pretendinous band, but comes to lie medial to the lateral digital sheet as the spiral band passes under the neurovascular bundle to join the web space coalescence, affords the opportunity for a potentially dangerous situation for the surgeon: the spiral nerve. Whereas in normal anatomy the path of the neurovascular bundle is straight, and the fascial bands spiral around the nerve, as the bands contract into cords, their course becomes straight, forcing the nerve to spiral around the cord. The nerve is displaced medially and superficially; the thicker the cord, the more displacement in each direction (**Figs. 10** and **11**). Unfortunately, adding to the confusion over nomenclature, this thickened cord is named the spiral cord, although in fact its course is straight; it is the nerve that spirals around the cord. The spiral cord is the end result of thickening and shortening of the spiral band (which was also straight), the web space coalescence of Leibovic, the lateral digital sheet and Grayson ligament. The distal termination of the spiral cord is usually via Grayson ligament attachments to the periosteum and flexor sheath of the middle phalanx; hence,

its contracture can also lead to flexion of the MP and PIP joints. Increasing PIP flexion will result in proximal displacement of the most vulnerable location of the nerve, where it lies closest to the skin surface.

Spiral cords also occur in different circumstances. Thoma and Karpinski[15] described 2 types of cords originating from the fascia or tendon of the intrinsic muscles in the middle and ring fingers. In type 1 (**Fig. 12**), a lateral digital cord originates from the lumbrical or interosseous and inserts into the periosteum of the middle phalanx. The investigators state that this cord can cause contracture of only the PIP joint, although the investigators would have expected contracture of the MP joint as well, given the volar position of the intrinsic tendons at the MP joint. In type 2, the lumbrical or interosseous contributes to a spiral cord, causing displacement of the neurovascular bundle. Theirs was the first study to show that intrinsic muscle fascia or tendon can serve as origin for Dupuytren cords in fingers other than the small finger. Meathrel and Thoma[16] reported 27% incidence of intrinsic muscle involvement in diseased tissue.

Strickland and Bassett[17] described the "isolated digital cord" with origin from the periosteum at the base of the proximal phalanx and the musculotendinous junction of the intrinsic muscle. It coursed in an oblique direction, displacing the nerve as the cord straightened and thickened, inserting into the base of the middle phalanx. Spiral cords and isolated digital cords follow a similar course: at the middle of the proximal phalanx they lie dorsal to the neurovascular bundle, and as they pass from dorsal to volar they displace the neurovascular bundle medially.

Hettiaratchy and colleagues[18] reported double spiral nerves in 5 cases, which spiral a full 720° around diseased cords. They theorized that the proximal spiral results from the customary straightening of the pretendinous cord–spiral cord–web space coalescence-lateral digital sheet, and that the distal spiral results from straightening of cords composed of the pretendinous cord connecting with the lateral digital sheet, the retrovascular cord of Thomine, and Cleland ligaments.

In summary, these studies outline a number of scenarios in which the nerve assumes an unexpected position due to the contracture and thickening of adjacent pathologic cords. Given the potential danger of encountering a spiral nerve during treatment of Dupuytren disease, a reliable method to predict its existence is desirable. Umlas and colleagues[19] investigated the observation of a soft mass between the distal palmar crease and the proximal digital crease in each finger and its

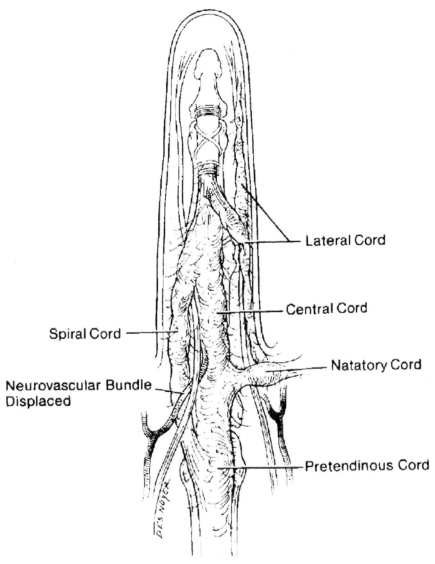

Fig. 10. Various pathologic cords in the finger and their locations. (*From* Strickland JW, Leibovic SJ. Anatomy and pathogenesis of the digital cords and nodules. Hand Clin 1991;7(4):645–57; with permission.)

relation to the presence of a spiral nerve. Although not the first to point out this association, Umlas and colleagues[19] showed that a combination of this mass and a PIP joint contracture was highly specific (94%) but not very sensitive (50%) at predicting the presence of a spiral nerve. They established that the presence of these 2 findings could be relied on to warn the surgeon of the presence of the spiral nerve, but its absence should not be seen as an indicator of safety.

Barton[20] and White[12] observed examples where Dupuytren tissue originated from the abductor digiti quinti fascia or tendon, and they both remarked on the difficulty in distinguishing the origins of cords in many circumstances in which they had thickened and caused a blending of adjacent fascial structures. It is sometimes impossible to discern the normal fascial origins of Dupuytren tissue when faced with a thickened, tight, dense collection of diseased tissue. It is not realistic to suppose that during surgery for Dupuytren contracture one can accurately identify the normal fascial precursor of all Dupuytren tissue. Use of the term "web space coalescence" by Strickland and Leibovic[9] was a validation of the observation that one cannot always define with accuracy the individual components of a mass of Dupuytren tissue. The fibers are densely interwoven in a chaotic pattern, defying individual identification.

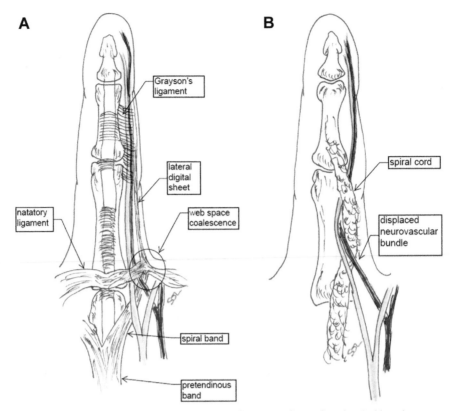

Fig. 11. (*A*) In normal anatomy, there is continuity among the pretendinous band, spiral band, natatory ligament, and lateral digital sheet. These structures all coalesce in the web space coalescence of Leibovic, shown in the circle. The spiral band passes under (deep to) the neurovascular bundle, so that although the proximal part of the spiral band is medial (with respect to the finger) to the bundle, the lateral digital sheet is lateral to the bundle. (*B*) The spiral cord displaces the neurovascular bundle as it contracts and straightens. The spiral cord is made up of diseased structures including the pretendinous band, spiral band, web space coalescence, lateral digital sheet, and Grayson ligament. (*Courtesy of* S. Leibovic, MD, Richmond, VA.)

Other regions coalesce as well. White[12] found that various parts of the fascia comingle and coalesce: on the ulnar side of the small finger, Grayson ligaments were continuous with the ulnar termination of the superficial transverse palmar ligament and a slip of the tendon of the abductor digiti quinti, whereas Cleland ligaments were continuous with fibers from the pretendinous band of the small finger and the lateral digital sheet, which also merged with the tendon of the abductor digiti quinti. Even the tendons of the abductor digiti quinti and the flexor digiti minimi were difficult to separate and distinguish from each other. The insertion site of the small finger cord will determine whether the PIP and/or DIP joints are contracted, as the cord may terminate with attachment to the middle phalanx base or shaft, distal phalanx base, or some combination of these locations.

The septae of Legueu and Juvara are involved in Dupuytren disease less frequently than the pretendinous bands. They are in close proximity to the spiral bands, flexor tendons, and neurovascular bundles, originating on the deep surface of the pretendinous bands and the palmar aponeurosis. Bilderback and Rayan[21] demonstrated thickening of the septae with Dupuytren disease as they coursed toward the web space coalescence, to which they contribute fibers. In surgical excision of Dupuytren disease, the existence of thickening in the septae of Legueu and Juvara is usually easily apparent. As the diseased tissue is raised and excised, from proximal to distal or from distal to proximal, extensions deep toward the flexor sheaths and metacarpals are readily apparent where they exist.

Contractures around the thumb and the first web space have a different pattern than in the fingers. The most common cord associated with the thumb is a thickening of the radial extension of the superficial transverse palmar ligament (also known as the proximal commissural ligament). By contrast, the ulnar portion of the superficial

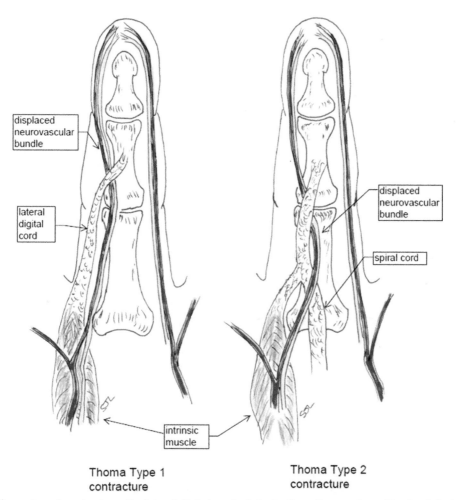

Thoma Type 1
contracture

Thoma Type 2
contracture

Fig. 12. Thoma type 1 contracture: the lateral digital cord originates from the muscle and fascia of the lumbrical muscle. Thoma and Karpinski[15] describes contracture of PIP joint only, although one would expect contraction of the MP joint as well with this configuration. Thoma type 2 contracture: the pathologic cord is made up of a cord from the intrinsic muscle as well as the pretendinous cord. It is a typical spiral cord with additional contribution from the intrinsic muscle fascia. It leads to both PIP and MP contractures. (*Courtesy of* S. Leibovic, MD, Richmond, VA.)

transverse palmar ligament, from the index ray and continuing ulnarly, is not often involved in thickening or contracture. The radial extension of the natatory ligament also can be involved (also known as the distal commissural ligament) in the first web space. Fibers from both the radial extension of the superficial transverse palmar ligament and the radial extension of the natatory ligament also may terminate in the skin of the first web space and of the thumb. The thumb is the fourth most commonly involved ray in Dupuytren contracture, after the ring, small, and middle fingers.[22] Dupuytren disease in the first web space may cause no contracture and be asymptomatic, although as it contracts, it can limit both radial and palmar abduction of the thumb. The thumb

does not often have a pretendinous band, although if it does and it becomes diseased, it may cause thumb MP contracture.

Anatomy may shed light on the relative incidence of Dupuytren contracture in the digits. Lanting and colleagues[22] studied the relative prevalence of Dupuytren contracture in each of the fingers in a sample of 344 Dutch hands. Most commonly affected was the ring finger, followed by the small and middle fingers, the thumb, and the index finger. They also analyzed the prevalence of Dupuytren contracture occurring in pairs of fingers. They found that its occurrence on the ulnar side of the hand in the ring and small fingers had no correlation with its occurrence on the radial side in the index and middle fingers. The most frequent pairs of fingers involved were the middle and ring, followed by the ring and small. It is known that the pretendinous bands send longitudinal fibers to the skin as their most superficial layer. These fibers are most prominent in the middle and ring fingers, and this is postulated as a reason why the simultaneous incidence in middle and ring fingers is highest. These fibers are also known to be common in the small finger, which may help explain their observed relatively high incidence of involvement of the middle, ring, and small fingers together.

Each of the cords described may cause contracture of specific joints as the cord shortens. Most commonly, the MP joints are contracted when the pretendinous cord is involved. The spiral cord, central cord, and the lateral digital cord type 1 of Thoma cause contraction of only the PIP joints. The isolated digital cord and lateral cord can cause contraction of only the DIP joints. Various other cords can cause contracture of 2 contiguous joints, as shown in **Table 2**. Some believe that the retrovascular cord of Thomine, the pathologic cord formed from the retrovascular band, may cause contracture of both the PIP and DIP joints.[8] Others believe that it affects only the PIP joint,[13] that it cannot cause a contracture, but failure to release it may prevent PIP joint contracture release. It is noted here that this distinction is confusing; it is not clear in Dupuytren disease how a cord can maintain a contracture but have no role in causing the contracture.

ANATOMY: A FINAL CONSIDERATION

In the past decade, treatments for Dupuytren contracture other than open fasciectomy have become more popular; yet, understanding the

Table 2
Cords and the joints they contract

Cord	Origin	Insertion	Joints Affected
Pretendinous cord	Palmar aponeurosis	Spiral cords	MP joint
Lateral digital cord, Thoma type 1	Lumbrical or interosseous	Base or shaft of middle phalanx	PIP joint only
Lateral digital cord, Thoma type 2	Lumbrical or interosseous and base of proximal phalanx, spiral band	Base or shaft of middle phalanx, lateral digital sheet, Grayson ligament	MP and PIP joint
Spiral cord	Pretendinous band, spiral band, web space coalescence	Web space coalescence, lateral digital sheet, Grayson ligaments	PIP joint
Central cord	Extension of pretendinous cord	Flexor sheath near PIP joint, or periosteum of middle phalanx	PIP joint
Isolated digital cord	Periosteum, base of proximal phalanx, abductor digiti quinti fascia or tendon	Periosteum and tendon sheath, middle phalanx; sometimes to distal phalanx	PIP joint, possibly DIP joint
Lateral cord	Lateral digital sheet	Skin or flexor sheath over middle phalanx and distally, Grayson ligaments	PIP joint, possibly DIP joint
Retrovascular cord of Thomine	Periosteum of proximal phalanx	Periosteum of distal phalanx	DIP joint, PIP joint or both DIP and PIP joints (debated)
Natatory ligament, extension to thumb	Natatory ligament	Skin of first web space, thumb proximal phalanx and flexor sheath	First web space
Superficial transverse palmar ligament, extension to thumb	Superficial transverse palmar ligament in palm	Skin of first web space and at base of thumb	First web space

Abbreviations: DIP, distal interphalangeal; MP, metacarpophalangeal; PIP, proximal interphalangeal.

anatomy of Dupuytren cords and nodules is no less important than in the past, to prevent damage to normal structures during treatment. Nodules, often the first stage of the disease, can arise de novo in otherwise normal tissue, usually between the superficial palmar fascia and the skin. They may represent metaplasia of fibro-fatty tissue normally present in these locations. As the disease progresses, cords form in predictable locations throughout the hand. We have seen that these locations follow the paths of normal anatomic structures, although they deform themselves, as well as adjacent normal structures, as they thicken and contract. Therefore, knowledge of these paths is critical to prevent damage during treatment of Dupuytren contracture.

The author believes that to subscribe exclusively to the extrinsic theory, that cords and nodules arise de novo in undiseased normal tissue, perilously ignores the observation that cords clearly follow definable paths derived from the known course of normal fascial bands. Similarly, blind acceptance of the intrinsic theory, wherein cords and nodules are believed to all arise in and from normal undiseased fascial structures, ignores the randomness of locations for nodules. Therefore, as Gosset[10] described, the locations of diseased tissue in Dupuytren contracture are best explained by a synthesis of both the intrinsic and extrinsic theory, as described herein. Furthermore, the author has attempted to harmonize the conflicting nomenclature and terminology for both (normal) bands and (diseased) cords, summarized in **Table 1**, to promote understanding and uniformity in descriptions of the disease process.

REFERENCES

1. Ketchum LD. The rationale for treating the nodule in Dupuytren's disease. Plast Reconstr Surg Glob Open 2014;2:e278, 1–11.
2. Murrell GAC. The role of the fibroblast in Dupuytren's contracture. Hand Clin 1991;7(4):669–80.
3. Badalamente MA, Hurst LC. The biochemistry of Dupuytren's disease. Hand Clin 1999;15(1):35–42.
4. Tomasek JJ, Vaughan MB, Haaksma CJ. Cellular structure and biology of Dupuytren's disease. Hand Clin 1999;15(1):21–34.
5. MacCallum P, Hueston JT. The pathology of Dupuytren's contracture. Aust N Z J Surg 1962;31:241–53.
6. McFarlane RM. Patterns of the diseased fascia in the fingers of Dupuytren's contracture. Plast Reconstr Surg 1974;54:31–44.
7. McFarlane RM. The anatomy of Dupuytren's disease. In: Hueston JT, Tubiana R, editors. Dupuytren's disease. London: Churchill Livingstone; 1985. p. 55–72.
8. McFarlane RM. Dupuytren's disease. In: McCarthy JG, May JW, Littler JW, editors. Plastic surgery. Philadelphia: W.B. Saunders; 1990. p. 5053–86.
9. Strickland JW, Leibovic SJ. Anatomy and pathogenesis of the digital cords and nodules. Hand Clin 1991;7(4):645–57.
10. Gosset J. Dupuytren's disease and the anatomy of the palmodigital aponeuroses. In: Hueston JT, Tubiana R, editors. Dupuytren's disease. London: Churchill Livingstone; 1985. p. 13–26.
11. Holland AJA, McGrouther DA. Clin Anat 1997;10: 97–103.
12. White S. Anatomy of the palmar fascia on the ulnar border of the hand. J Hand Surg Br 1984;9(1):50–6.
13. Rayan GM. Dupuytren disease: anatomy, pathology, presentation and treatment. J Bone Joint Surg Am 2007;89(1):190–8.
14. Zdilla MJ. The hand of sabazios: evidence of Dupuytren's disease in antiquity and the origin of the hand of benediction. J Hand Surg Asian Pac Vol 2017;22(3):403–40.
15. Thoma A, Karpinski M. Involvement of the interosseous and lumbrical muscle-tendon units in the lateral and spiral cords in Dupuytren's disease of the middle fingers. Plast Reconstr Surg 2017;140: 116–24.
16. Meathrel KE, Thoma A. Abductor digiti minimi involvement in Dupuytren's contracture of the small finger. J Hand Surg Am 2004;29(3):510–3.
17. Strickland JW, Basset RL. The isolated digital cord in Dupuytren's contractures: anatomy and clinical significance. J Hand Surg Am 1985;10(1):118–24.
18. Hettiaratchy S, Tonkin MA, Edmunds IA. Spiralling of the neurovascular bundle in Dupuytren's disease. J Hand Surg Eur Vol 2010;35(2):103–8.
19. Umlas ME, Bischoff RJ, Gelberman RH. Predictors of neurovascular displacement in hands with Dupuytren's contracture. J Hand Surg Br 1994;19(1): 664–6.
20. Barton NJ. Dupuytren's disease arising from the abductor digiti minimi. J Hand Surg Br 1984;9(3): 265–70.
21. Bilderback KK, Rayan GM. Dupuytren's cord involving the septa of Legueu and Juvara: a case report. J Hand Surg Am 2002;27(2):344–6.
22. Lanting S, Nooraee N, Werker PMN, et al. Patterns of Dupuytren disease in fingers: studying correlations with a multivariate ordinal logit model. Plast Reconstr Surg 2014;134:483–90.

Needle Aponeurotomy for Dupuytren Disease

Kate E. Elzinga, MD, FRCSC[a], Michael J. Morhart, MD, MS, FRCSC[b],*

KEYWORDS

- Dupuytren disease • Needle aponeurotomy • Fasciectomy • Collagenase injection

KEY POINTS

- Needle aponeurotomy is an effective, minimally invasive treatment for metacarpophalangeal and interphalangeal joint contractures caused by Dupuytren disease. Multiple joints and digits can be safely treated in 1 session.
- Needle aponeurotomy is more cost-effective and has a significantly lower rate of complications compared with open fasciectomy and collagenase injections.
- Recurrence rates for needle aponeurotomy are higher compared with open fasciectomy and collagenase injections.
- Patient satisfaction rates are very high following needle aponeurotomy; the single clinic visit required and the minimal downtime after treatment are advantages unique to this procedure.

INTRODUCTION: NATURE OF THE PROBLEM

Dupuytren disease is a fibroproliferative disorder that can affect the fascia of the palmar wrist,[1] hand, and fingers, resulting in aesthetic and functional concerns for patients. Dupuytren disease has a 5% prevalence in the United States[2] and a 3% to 5% prevalence in the United Kingdom.[3] Dupuytren cords causing symptomatic digital flexion contractures can be treated with percutaneous needle aponeurotomy (NA), as described by Lermusiaux and Debeyre[4] in 1980 and Badois and colleagues[5] in 1993. Nearly all metacarpophalangeal (MCP) joint contractures can be fully corrected with 1 session of NA. Proximal interphalangeal (PIP) joint contractures can be more difficult to fully correct.[6] NA can be used as a primary treatment of Dupuytren contracture or to delay fasciectomy.[7]

From 2007 to 2014 in the United States, approximately 15% of patients treated for Dupuytren disease underwent NA.[8] This trend was consistent over time despite the introduction of collagenase *Clostridium histolyticum* injections in 2010.[8,9] Patient outcomes and satisfaction rates are similar for NA and collagenase.[10] Dermatofasciectomy, fasciectomy, and fasciotomy are alternative open treatments for Dupuytren contracture.

The advantages of NA compared with open fasciectomy include the single clinic visit required for the procedure, the avoidance of palmar incisions and the subsequent risk of flap necrosis and wound dehiscence, and a faster recovery (**Table 1**). Only small aliquots of local anesthesia are required, making the procedure safer, particularly for older patients with other comorbidities. The risks of infection, hematoma, and digital nerve injury are lower for NA compared with open fasciectomy.[11] Compared with collagenase injections, complication rates for NA are also significantly lower.[12] NA is significantly more cost-effective than open fasciectomy and collagenase injections.[12]

Disclosure: K.E. Elzinga has no disclosures. M.J. Morhart is a consultant for Actelion Pharmaceuticals Canada for the product Xiaflex.
[a] Section of Plastic Surgery, University of Calgary, 4448 Front Street Southeast, Calgary, Alberta T3M 1M4, Canada; [b] Division of Plastic Surgery, University of Alberta, 14310 111 Avenue Northwest, Edmonton, Alberta T5M 3Z7, Canada
* Corresponding author.
E-mail address: MMorhart@morhart.ca

Table 1
Advantages and disadvantages of various treatments for Dupuytren disease

	Open Fasciectomy	Needle Aponeurotomy	Collagenase *C histolyticum*
Advantages	• Direct visualization of the cord, flexor tendons, and neurovascular structures • Permits excision of the diseased palmar fascia	• Fast, minimally invasive procedure • Rapid recovery • Dressings only required if a skin tear occurs • Performed in a single clinic visit • Only subdermal, small-volume, local anesthetic is required • Hand therapy is rarely required • Least discomfort at treatment site[12] • Lowest rate of flare reactions and complex regional pain syndrome • Lower cost,[16] minimal equipment and nursing care required • Minimal time off work • Higher patient satisfaction than open fasciectomy[17,18]	• Fast, minimally invasive procedure • Rapid recovery • Dressings only required if skin tear occurs • Hand therapy is rarely required • Minimal time off work • High rate of patient satisfaction[19,20] • Lowest rate of digital nerve injury[21]
Disadvantages	• Most invasive procedure • Often performed in the operating room with regional or general anesthesia. However, can safely be performed using the WALANT technique[22] • Postoperative hand therapy typically required • Highest cost • Postoperative dressings required • Suture removal required (or time for absorbable sutures to break down) • Highest rate of wound complications (dehiscence, delayed healing, skin flap edge necrosis) • Highest rate of neurovascular injury, both temporary and permanent • Longest healing time • More painful compared with NA[17] • Postoperative scarring can lead to new contractures • Longer patient wait times[23] • More time off work	• Steep learning curve • Higher recurrence rate • Fastest time to recurrence • Higher rate of flexion tendon rupture than open fasciectomy	• Two clinic visits required per treatment • Digital or wrist nerve blocks required before manipulation • Multiple treatments can be required for optimal contracture correction and/or to treat multiple digits • Expensive • Increased discomfort following the procedure compared with NA • Physician or assistant expertise is required to prepare the collagenase for injection

Abbreviation: WALANT, wide-awake local anesthesia no tourniquet.

The main disadvantage of NA is its higher recurrence rate compared with open fasciectomy, particularly for younger patients (<35 years old) and for PIP joint contractures.[13] Based on our experience, we counsel patients that recurrence rates for open fasciectomy and collagenase are approximately 50% at 5 years, compared with 50% at 3 years for NA. If recurrence occurs, many patients choose to undergo repeat NA treatment. Repeat NA is straightforward and is not associated with increased complications.[14] Treatment with a third or fourth NA is equally effective as a primary or secondary NA.[15]

INDICATIONS/CONTRAINDICATIONS

Any symptomatic palpable cord can be treated with NA (**Table 2**); joint contractures do not need to attain a certain degree of impairment before treatment, unlike the current indications for open fasciectomy. Pretendinous, spiral, lateral, natatory, adductor, and retrovascular cords can be effectively treated with NA. Some investigators believe that treatment is most effective and long-lasting for patients treated with early contracture and minimal PIP joint arthrofibrosis.[24] NA can be performed for patients seeking their first Dupuytren treatment as well as those with a history of open fasciectomy, collagenase injection, or NA.

Patients without a palpable cord should not be treated with NA. Dupuytren nodules can be observed, treated with steroid injections if painful, or surgically excised.

SURGICAL TECHNIQUE/PROCEDURE
Preoperative Planning

The patient's medical and surgical history, medications, allergies, and smoking status are reviewed. Physical examination is performed, focusing on the hands. Documentation of neurovascular status; severity of skin involvement; and presence of cords, nodules, and skin dimpling is completed. Active and passive range of motion measurements are recorded for the MCP and interphalangeal (IP) joints of the bilateral hands. Photographs of the hands are taken before treatment and at subsequent follow-up appointments.

Treatment options are discussed with the patient, including observation, NA, collagenase injections, and open fasciectomy. Joint decision-making occurs between the hand surgeon and the patient to determine the preferred course of treatment. The authors favor NA rather than open fasciectomy given its low complication rate, rapid recovery, ease of scheduling in a clinic or office setting, avoidance of regional or general anesthesia, and low cost.

Smoking cessation is encouraged but is not an absolute contraindication for NA or collagenase injections. Open fasciectomy is not offered to smokers given the higher risk of skin flap necrosis, wound dehiscence, and anesthetic complications.

Anticoagulation is held before NA for low-risk patients. Patients at high risk of thrombosis are asked to continue their anticoagulation and are counseled about their higher risk of ecchymosis and hematoma following the procedure. Hematoma rates are lower for NA compared with open fasciectomy[11]; NA is our preferred treatment of anticoagulated patients.

Patients are counseled that they may experience some discomfort during NA. They are asked to communicate with their surgeons with respect to pain or paresthesias (Tinel sign) throughout the procedure and to avoid moving their hands.

Dupuytren Cord Assessment

When first starting to use the technique of NA, the authors recommend treating patients with a well-defined pretendinous cord causing an MCP joint contracture; these cords are the most easily and most safely treated with NA. As clinicians become more experienced, PIP cord contractures can be treated, noting that there is less distance between the cord and the flexor tendons below and the neurovascular bundles are in closer proximity over the proximal phalanx compared with in the palm. Abductor digiti minimi cords can be treated but require greater experience with the technique because of the proximity to the ulnar neurovascular bundle of the small finger.

The bevel of the needle is oriented perpendicular to the cord and used as a blade to sharply divide the cord with a gentle sweeping motion.

Table 2 Indications and relative contraindications for needle aponeurotomy for Dupuytren disease	
Indications	**Relative Contraindications**
Any symptomatic MCP or IP joint flexion contraction with a palpable cord	Aggressive disease with rapid recurrence following any previous treatment; consider dermatofasciectomy, arthrodesis, or ray amputation
Informed, cooperative patient	Severe skin shortage, scarring

Abbreviation: IP, interphalangeal.

For a pretendinous cord, the bevel points distal. For a first web space adductor cord or a natatory cord, the bevel points ulnar or radial. Because of the close proximity of the digital artery and nerve, the authors recommend caution when performing NA for a retrovascular cord causing a distal IP (DIP) joint contracture.

Care is taken to minimize the risk of laceration of the radial and ulnar neurovascular structures with NA. NA at the volar digital skin creases is avoided; the digital arteries and nerves are located closer to the skin in these areas. To maximize the distance between the Dupuytren cord and the flexor tendons below, NA is performed at locations of maximal bowstringing of the cord volarly. Midline division of the cord is preferred to minimize the risk to the neurovascular structures. For very thick, wide cords, 2 portals may be used side by side, a few millimeters apart. Because the neurovascular bundles can be displaced toward the midline and volarly by spiral cords, frequent communication with the patient is critical. If the patient reports any nerve irritation (electrical shocks, tingling, or other dysesthesias radiating over the ulnar or radial digit), the needle must be repositioned.

NA is most easily performed through supple, mobile, healthy skin. Working through Dupuytren nodules, previous surgical incisions, and skin grafts is possible but decreases the tactile difference typically felt between unscarred, supple skin and the thick, fibrous cord below.

Preparation and Patient Positioning

To maximize efficiency, minimize medical waste and cost, and improve patient satisfaction, NA is performed in a clinic or office procedure room without the need for sedation or tourniquet.[22] The patient is positioned supine on the bed with the affected hand out on an arm board. For wheelchair-bound patients and others with decreased mobility or the inability to lie flat because of back pain or other conditions, the procedure can be performed with the patient seated. The authors prefer to have the patient supine when possible to minimize light-headedness and apprehension.

Both hands can safely be treated at the same time but this can impair patient self-care following the procedure. Patients are counseled about the risk of a skin tear and the subsequent need for a daily dressing. After reviewing the expected postoperative course, they may choose to proceed with staged treatment or simultaneous treatment of bilateral hand Dupuytren contractures. If the patient chooses to have both hands treated during the same session, the authors treat the most

symptomatic hand first and then confirm whether the patient would like to proceed with the contralateral hand. If a skin tear occurs during treatment of the first hand, treatment of the second hand is delayed.

The NA treatment sites (portals) are marked using a fine marker (**Fig. 1**). The number of portals varies based on the cord, with longer and wider cords requiring more portals. In general, a minimum of 3 portals are used. Other surgeons have used an average of 1.8[25] to more than 10 portals per digit.[26] Ideally, portals are marked in areas of skin excess with good mobility. Scarred, tethered, and dimpled areas and skin flexion creases are avoided. The NA portals are marked over the center of the cord at intervals 5 mm apart or more. Two portals can be used for wide cords, with 1 portal over the radial aspect and another over the ulnar aspect of the cord, at the same level.

The patient's wrist, hand, and fingers are prepped using an antiseptic solution. A basic surgical tray is opened (**Fig. 2**). A sterile surgical towel is placed on the hand table; the patient's supinated hand is placed on it. A second towel is placed to cover the patient's volar wrist and forearm. A rolled surgical towel is placed under the dorsal MCP joints to facilitate MCP and PIP joint extension. Preoperative antibiotics are not indicated for NA; it is a clean, elective, outpatient hand procedure.[27–29]

Surgical Approach

1. Local anesthetic, typically 1% lidocaine, is injected in the immediate subdermal plane, creating a small skin bleb, at the NA portals, staying superficial to preserve sensory feedback from the radial and ulnar digital nerves below. A 1-mL syringe is used with a 12-mm (0.5 inch) 30-gauge needle. Approximately 0.1 mL is placed at each treatment portal.

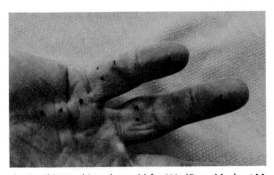

Fig. 1. Skin markings (portals) for NA. (*From* Morhart M. Pearls and pitfalls of needle aponeurotomy in Dupuytren's disease. Plast Reconstr Surg 2015;135(3):819; with permission.)

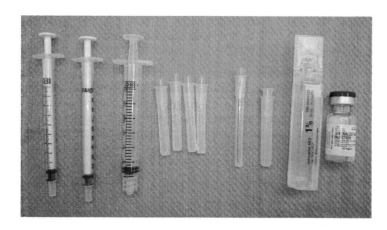

Fig. 2. Equipment required for needle aponeurotomy. Two 1-mL syringes, a 3-mL syringe, four 25-gauge needles (number varies based on the disease treated; replace frequently because they dull easily), an 18-gauge needle, a 30-gauge needle, 1% lidocaine plain, and triamcinolone are used. (*From* Morhart M. Pearls and pitfalls of needle aponeurotomy in Dupuytren's disease. Plast Reconstr Surg 2015;135(3):818; with permission.)

The local anesthetic can be placed at all portals initially or sequentially as each portal is used; the authors recommend the latter approach for practitioners new to the procedure, because this facilitates adjustment of portals as the treatment progresses. The subdermal fat and Dupuytren cords are insensate.[30–32]

2. Short (16 mm [5/8 inch]) 25-gauge needles are used in most cases to perform NA. For thick cords, a 20-gauge or 18-gauge needle can be used. The needles are changed frequently to maintain a sharp cutting bevel tip. The authors prefer to attach the needle to a 1-mL syringe; others prefer to hold the needle alone.

3. Treatment progresses from distal to proximal, with the goal of releasing the cord sequentially at each marked NA portal. The PIP joint is released first, followed by the MCP joint. The portals can be adjusted as necessary during the procedure.

4. Using the contralateral hand, the surgeon applies traction to the volar skin just distal to the portal being treated. The traction aids in stabilizing the treatment site and is performed throughout the procedure. Care is taken to avoid extending the finger to prevent movement of the flexor tendons closer to the volar skin, putting them at higher risk of injury, particularly when releasing MCP joint contractures. Some extension can be used while releasing PIP joint contractures; the pulleys limit flexor tendon bowstringing more in the digit compared with in the palm.

5. The cord is palpated and its three-dimensional nature is mentally visualized by the surgeon. The needle is introduced perpendicularly into the center of the cord through the most distal portal. The needle is felt entering the cord. The patient is asked to flex the finger; if the needle

moves, it has been inserted too deeply, penetrating the flexor tendon, and must be withdrawn into the substance of the cord. Excessive sharp pain, particularly during each sweep of the needle, may be an indication that the needle has penetrated the flexor tendon sheath or pulley system; patients are asked to communicate any increased discomfort to the surgeon.

6. Once appropriately located within the cord, the needle is moved radially and ulnarly in smooth sweeping motions like a pendulum, from superficial to deep, incrementally, to release the cord. The cord feels gritty and a grating sound can be heard as it is sharply released. If there is no resistance, the needle is not appropriately placed in the cord and should be repositioned. Once the cord's resistance is lost, and a soft spot can be palpated, the next portal is addressed.

7. Patients are asked frequently whether they feel any paresthesias indicating the needle's proximity to a digital nerve and thus the need to relocate the needle. Light touch sensation to the ulnar and radial volar distal phalanx is reassessed before treatment at each portal. If an injury to a proper digital nerve is suspected, the NA procedure is stopped, a digital block is placed, and the finger is opened. The nerve is explored. If lacerated, it is repaired using microsurgical technique with 9-0 nylon suture.

8. For Dupuytren skin pitting, the needle is used to sweep under the dermis, creating a plane between the skin and the nodule below. This maneuver decreases the skin tethering and chance of a skin tear. An 18-gauge needle can be helpful for performing this subdermal horizontal release, also known as a dermolysis or subcision.[33]

9. After cutting through the cord at each subsequent level, the finger is extended. This extension is particularly helpful for pretendinous cords. An audible pop can often be heard as the cord is fully released. Firm digital pressure over the portal site after NA is another technique for final separation of the cord. Gentle massaging is very helpful for natatory cords.

10. After performing NA at each of the portals, the finger is reassessed (**Figs. 3** and **4**). Once the predominant cord has been released, lesser cords may become palpable on the other side of the digit. These lesser cords are marked with a sterile marker and further NA is performed until all palpable cords have been released and optimal passive extension is achieved.

11. A digital block can be performed after NA to permit final passive stretching of the digit and final correction of joint contractures. Closed capsulotomy for residual PIP flexion contractures can be performed. Steroids are injected to promote endogenous collagenase activity. Triamcinolone degrades insoluble collagen to salt-soluble collagen, which can then be excreted by the body.[34,35] The authors use a 3-mL syringe containing 2.5 mL of 1% lidocaine and 0.5 mL of 40 mg/mL (ie, 20 mg) triamcinolone (Sandoz Canada Inc., Boucherville, Quebec) for each digit. We inject along the digit, in each of the portals, in the subcutaneous tissues. We aim to extend the MCP joints to approximately 10°

of hyperextension and the PIP joints to neutral, while keeping the wrist flexed to minimize tension on the flexor tendons.

Our operative time averages 15 minutes per digit treated. The authors treat all palpable cords of the hand in 1 session, aiming for full release of all contractures. We typically recommend staged treatment of the hands to the patient but have performed bilateral hand releases in more than 50 patients with no adverse outcomes.

Corticosteroids

McMillan and Binhammer[36] showed a significantly greater correction of flexion contractures at 6 months for patients treated with NA combined with triamcinolone steroid injections (87% correction) than with NA alone (64% improvement) in their randomized controlled trial. They injected the cords directly after NA using 8 to 48 mg of triamcinolone per digit (mean, 42 mg), up to 120 mg per hand based on the extent of the disease. Repeat injections were performed at 6 weeks (mean, 34 mg) and 3 months (mean, 24 mg) after NA when areas of palpable thickness were present along previously released cords.

Lipofilling

Lipofilling in combination with NA was described by Hovius and colleagues[37] in 2011. The investigators used regional or general anesthesia, upper extremity exsanguination and tourniquet, a lead hand

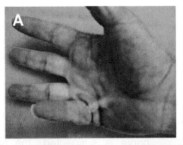
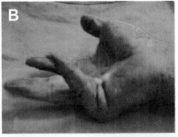
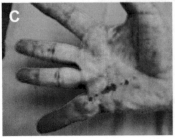
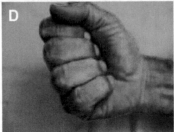
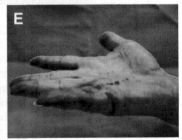

Fig. 3. (*A, B*) Before and (*C–E*) after needle aponeurotomy for a small finger MCP joint flexion contracture. (*Adapted from* Morhart M. Pearls and pitfalls of needle aponeurotomy in Dupuytren's disease. Plast Reconstr Surg 2015;135(3):821; with permission.)

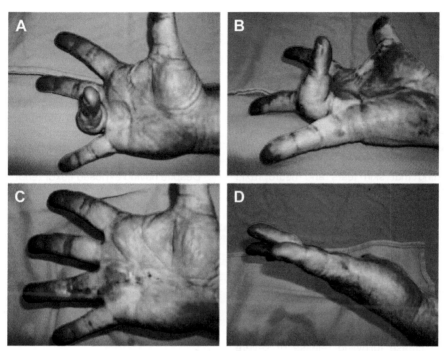

Fig. 4. (*A, B*) Before and (*C, D*) after needle aponeurotomy for a ring finger PIP joint flexion contracture. (*Adapted from* Morhart M. Pearls and pitfalls of needle aponeurotomy in Dupuytren's disease. Plast Reconstr Surg 2015;135(3):822; with permission.)

retractor, extensive frequent placement of the needle to severe the cord superficially along its course (up to 50 punctures per digit), a Dupuytome (Marina Medical, Sunrise, FL) L-shaped cutting device for skin pits, lipofilling (10 mL of fat placed per digit on average), and an extension splint for 1 week postoperatively followed by nighttime splinting for 3 to 6 months. Operative time was 1 to 1.5 hours. For the 50 patients studied, at a mean follow-up of 44 weeks, the MCP joint flexion contractures had improved from 37° to −5° and the PIP joint flexion contractures from 61° to 27°. Complications included 1 digital nerve injury, 1 wound infection, and 4 cases of complex regional pain syndrome.

In 2016, the same group published their 1-year results for patients undergoing NA with lipofilling in a prospective randomized controlled trial compared with patients undergoing limited fasciectomy.[38] They concluded that NA with lipofilling had a faster recovery (return to normal daily activities at 9 days for NA and lipofilling, 19 days for fasciectomy), similar efficacy (18% for NA with lipofilling, 9% for fasciectomy), and fewer complications (5% of patients developed complex regional pain syndrome after NA and lipofilling, 3% developed complex regional pain syndrome and 6% sustained a neurovascular injury after fasciectomy) compared with open fasciectomy.

Patient satisfaction was higher in the NA and lipofilling group. They did not compare their technique with NA alone.

Ultrasonography

Sakellariou and colleagues[39] described the technique of ultrasonography-assisted NA. This technique may be particularly useful for hand surgeons with expertise in ultrasonography imaging while learning the technique of NA. Ultrasonography provides additional information about the location of the neurovascular bundles and flexor tendons.[14] It can provide reassurance that the treatment portals have been safely marked. Using ultrasonography increases the treatment time and cost. The authors believe that direct tactile feedback provides the highest patient safety rather than relying on radiologic modalities.

COMPLICATIONS AND MANAGEMENT

The senior author has performed more than 2000 NAs over the past 10 years in an outpatient clinic. Patient satisfaction rates are high and complication rates have been low. The most common complication is a skin tear, occurring in 5% of cases. There have been 2 acute flexor tendon ruptures (both while treating small finger PIP joint contractures), no delayed flexor tendon ruptures, no cases of complex regional pain syndrome, and no permanent injuries to the digital neurovascular structures. Transient neuropraxias have occurred in 2% to 5% of patients and have resolved spontaneously within 3 months.

Complications rates have been reported to occur in up to 67% of patients undergoing open fasciectomy, most commonly consisting of nerve injury, infection, and complex regional pain syndrome (**Table 3**).[40] In contrast, Pess and colleagues[13] reported on 1013 digits treated with NA, indicating that skin tears and neuropraxia were the most common complications, occurring in 3% and 1% of patients, respectively. One digital nerve injury occurred. No tendon ruptures, cases of complex regional pain syndrome, or infections were reported.

Skin Tear

Skin tears occur in 5% of our patients; other have reported rates of 3% to 68%.[13,14,17,26,52] Most tears occur at the base of the finger in the MCP joint flexion crease following release of severe flexion contractures. Tears are also common where the skin is adherent to the underlying cord; we attempt to minimize tears at these areas by using a needle to release the skin from the cord below (dermolysis/subcision) before extending the finger. Releasing the cord at multiple levels before full gentle extension of the digit decreases tearing.

If a skin tear does occur, pressure is applied to the wound using a gauze until the bleeding slows. Then a dressing is applied using white petroleum (Vaseline), gauze, and Coban tape. The patient is taught that a moist wound environment improves healing and is shown how to perform a dressing change daily.[53] A previous randomized controlled study of 922 patients demonstrated that white petroleum is safe and effective with an equally low rate of infection and a lower incidence of allergic contact dermatitis compared with bacitracin.[54] Sterile dressings are not required; clean dressings are sufficient and minimize patient costs.[55] Patients are encouraged to do active range of motion multiple times daily during the healing phase to prevent stiffness.

Despite having exposed flexor tendons, pulleys, and neurovascular structures, secondary healing occurs promptly. Most skin tears heal within 2 to 3 weeks (**Fig. 5**). Primary closure, skin grafts, and local flaps are not indicated.

Skin tears are also common following treatment with collagenase. Grandizio and colleagues[56] reported a 24% incidence of skin tears following collagenase treatment of MCP and PIP joint contractures, which correlated with the degree of the contracture.

Infection

Patients with skin tears can experience mild erythema surrounding their wounds as healing progresses, caused by increases in local blood flow. Routine antibiotics are not necessary for patients with skin tears. The authors have had 1 case of cellulitis that resolved with oral antibiotics. No cases of flexor tenosynovitis have been observed by our group, although rare cases have been reported in the literature. Herrera and colleagues[26] reported 2 cases in their series of 525 digits treated with NA.

Table 3 Complication rates following treatment of Dupuytren disease			
	Primary Open Fasciectomy (%)	Needle Aponeurotomy (%)	Collagenase C histolyticum (%)
Digital nerve injury	3.4[41]	0.1–4[13,42,43]	NR
Neuropraxia	0.4–46[44]	1–6[45]	NR
Arterial injury	2[41]	0[13]	1 case reported[46]
Wound healing complications	22.9[41]	3–50[17,32,42,47]	11–34[32,48]
Hematoma	2.1[41]	0.3[42]	51[49]
Complex regional pain syndrome	5.8[40,41,50]	0[13]	1[40]
Skin tears	NR	3.4[13]	9–15[40]
Flexor tendon injury	NR	0.05[42]	0.27[51]
Infection	2.4[41]	0.7[42]	NR[49]

Abbreviation: NR, not reported.
Adapted from Cheung K, Walley KC, Rozental TD. Management of complications of Dupuytren contracture. Hand Clin 2015;31(2):348; with permission.

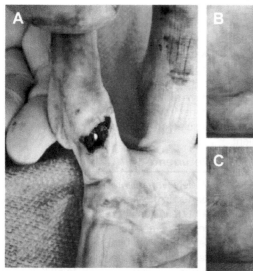
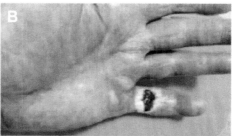
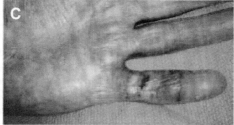

Fig. 5. Skin tears that occur during needle aponeurotomy heal well by secondary intention, as shown here with exposure of the flexor tendons. Note the healing of the small finger tear, (A) shown immediately after finger extension manipulation, (B) 8 days after needle aponeurotomy, and (C) 18 days after needle aponeurotomy. (*Adapted from* Morhart M. Pearls and pitfalls of needle aponeurotomy in Dupuytren's disease. Plast Reconstr Surg 2015;135(3):823; with permission.)

Bleeding

Patients on anticoagulation who experience skin tears are taught how to apply direct pressure if new bleeding is noted at home following NA. To date, the authors have not had any patients report complications caused by bleeding, whether anticoagulated or not.

Flexor Tendon Rupture

The authors have experienced 2 small finger zone 2 flexor tendon ruptures acutely during NA early in our NA experience. Both were repaired immediately. One percent lidocaine with epinephrine was injected as a digital block. Tendon repair was performed wide-awake with no tourniquet using a 6-strand core suture technique followed by an epitendinous suture. The patients were asked to flex and extend their fingers to assess for tendon gapping and gliding at the time of repair; adjustments to tendon sutures and pulley venting are performed as indicated. Early active range of motion therapy is instituted. Patients are splinted to protect the flexor tendon repair between exercises. They are closely supervised by a hand therapist.

Other investigators report delayed tendon ruptures as patients use their hand actively several weeks after NA; the authors have not experienced this complication to date. Five cases of delayed flexor tendon rupture were reported out of 50,000 procedures by Lermusiaux and

colleagues.[6] Herrera and colleagues[26] reported 1 case out of 525 digits treated with NA.

POSTOPERATIVE CARE

Small, round, adhesive bandages are placed over each NA treatment site. Patients remove them at their discretion, within 24 hours of the procedure. Elevation and ice are encouraged for the first 48 hours. Patients may use their hands immediately for activities of daily living. Heavy grasping and sports are avoided for 1 week. Hand therapy is rarely necessary. No medications are prescribed; patients are advised to use over-the-counter acetaminophen and ibuprofen if needed for pain.

Routine splinting is not used. Ebskov and colleagues[57] found that dynamic extension splinting at night for at least 3 months did not alter the natural course of Dupuytren disease or lessen recurrence of contracture. Similarly, a multicenter, randomized controlled trial performed by Jerosch-Herold and colleagues[58] found no benefit of routine splinting. They concluded that splinting generated unnecessary expenses to the health care system and was inconvenient for patients. They recommended splinting only for patients with early recurrence of flexion contractures postoperatively.

However, for patients with full passive extension but an active extensor lag greater than 10° to 20° at the PIP joint after NA, the authors prescribe extension splinting and hand therapy. A boutonniere or a relative motion splint is made by a hand therapist for the PIP joint to encourage dorsal movement of the lateral bands with active DIP motion and gradual improvement of the central slip attenuation after correction of the prolonged PIP joint flexion. The splint is worn during the day and at night for 3 weeks and then continued at night only for 3 months. During the first 3 weeks, the splint is removed 5 times daily by the patient and passive and active range of motion exercises are performed, under the guidance of a hand therapist. Active extensor lags less than 10° to 20° typically correct spontaneously over time.

OUTCOMES

Pess and colleagues[13] reported a 99% correction rate for MCP joint contractures and 89% for PIP joint contractions using NA for 1013 fingers (**Table 4**). Herrera and colleagues[26] reported a 98% correction rate for MCP joint contractures (total passive extension deficit improvement from 41° to 1°) with an 81% correction maintained at the 4.5-month follow-up and a 92% correction at the PIP joint with a 58% correction maintained at the 4.5-month follow-up for 525 digits.

Repeat NA can be performed with no increase in complications compared with the initial NA, which is in contrast with repeat open fasciectomy, for which complications rates are markedly higher for repeat treatment. Rates of digital nerve and artery injury have been reported at 3.1% and 1.7% respectively for primary open fasciectomy compared with 17% and 25.7% for repeat open fascicectomy.[41]

Flexion deficits are possible after any hand surgery, resulting in the inability to make a full fist. van Rijssen and colleagues[17] reported that, 6 weeks following Dupuytren treatment, 19 of 57 hands treated with limited fasciectomy had flexion deficits; these deficits were not present preoperatively. However, none of the 60 hands treated with NA developed flexion deficits. Patients treated with NA had higher satisfaction rates than those treated with fasciectomy. Scores on the disability of the arm, shoulder, and hand (DASH) questionnaire took longer to return to normal and complications rates were higher for patients in the fasciectomy group compared with the NA group.

Recurrence

Widely variable recurrence rates have been reported in the literature, in part because of inconsistent definitions of recurrence, variable methods of reporting, and variable use of goniometry.[59] A systematic review by Chen and colleagues[40] reported recurrence rates ranging from 0% to 39% for open partial fasciectomy, 50% to 58% for NA, and 10% to 31% for collagenase injection over variable follow-up intervals, up to 7 years. Rahr and colleagues[60] found that recurrence after NA was lower in patients with a total passive extension deficit less than 90° than in those with more severe contractures.

Various groups have found different factors to be associated with recurrence. For instance, Hindocha and colleagues[61] found that patients with all features of Dupuytren diathesis (family history [siblings/parents], bilateral Dupuytren disease, Garrod pads, male gender, age of onset <50 years old) had a 71% recurrence rate, whereas those with none of these risk factors had a recurrence rate of 23%. However, van Rijssen and colleagues[62] found that only younger age correlated with a higher recurrence rate.

Following all treatments, recurrence rates are higher for PIP joint contractures compared with MCP joint flexion contractures (**Table 5**). When in flexion, the collateral ligaments of the MCP joints are elongated but those of the PIP joint are

Table 4
Outcomes following needle aponeurotomy for Dupuytren disease

	Immediate Postoperative Result	Final Follow-up Result (3–6.2 y Postoperatively)
MCP joint contracture correction	• Average contracture improvement from 35° to 1° • 99% improvement	• Recurrent contracture 11° • 72% improvement maintained
PIP joint contracture correction	• Average contracture improvement from 50° to 6° • 89% improvement	• Recurrent contracture 35° • 31% improvement maintained

Total of 1013 fingers treated; minimum initial contracture of 20° or greater.
Data from Pess GM, Pess RM, Pess RA. Results of needle aponeurotomy for Dupuytren contracture in over 1000 fingers. J Hand Surg Am 2012;37(4):651–6.

Table 5
Recurrence rates following various treatments for Dupuytren contracture

	Overall Recurrence Rate (%)	MCP Joint (%)	PIP Joint (%)
Primary open fasciectomy	21[62]	21[62]	21[62]
Needle aponeurotomy	85[62]	57[62]	70[62]
Collagenase C histolyticum	35[63]	27[63]	56[63]

Adapted from Cheung K, Walley KC, Rozental TD. Management of complications of Dupuytren contracture. Hand Clin 2015;31(2):350; with permission.

shortened. Despite release of a Dupuytren cord causing a PIP flexion contracture, the tight, shortened collateral ligaments persist. The authors have had to treat 10 patients with PIP joint flexion contractures resistant to NA and closed capsulotomy with open surgery.

The randomized, prospective study of 115 hands by van Rijssen and colleagues[62] revealed a recurrence rate (defined as a worsening of the total passive extension deficit of 30°) of 85% following NA and 21% following limited fasciectomy at 5 years; this is the highest recurrence rate for NA reported to date. Steroids were not used during their NA treatment. For patients with recurrence following either NA or fasciectomy, most patients chose NA (4 of 9 patients after NA, 26 of 45 patients after fasciectomy) or no treatment (5 of 9 patients after NA, 12 of 45 patients after fasciectomy). The remaining 7 patients in the fasciectomy group chose repeat fasciectomy. Despite recurrence, patients are generally happy with NA and often choose NA again for treatment.

A single-blinded, prospective, randomized control trial by Strömberg and colleagues[64] concluded that treatment outcomes for MCP joint contractures with NA or collagenase were not significantly different at 1-year follow-up. Ninety percent of patients in both groups had maintained full extension of the treated MCP at 1 year. The cost of equipment to treat a patient with NA (material + local anesthetic + steroids = US$20) was significantly less than for collagenase (collagenase = US$730). Furthermore, NA patients only required 1 treatment visit, whereas collagenase patients required 2. Similarly, Scherman and colleagues[25] found NA and collagenase injections resulted in equal outcomes at 1 year for patients with primarily MCP joint contractures. Seventy percent improvement

was maintained at 1 year for both groups. A randomized controlled trial by Skov and colleagues[12] comparing collagenase injections with NA for isolated PIP joint contractures concluded that collagenase is not superior to NA and had a higher complication rate.

Patient Satisfaction

Zhou and colleagues[65] studied outcomes for patients with mild-moderate Dupuytren disease (Tubiana stage I–II, total passive extension deficit up to 90°; these stages account for 75% of with Dupuytren based on a review of 3357 patient charts[66]) (**Fig. 6**) at 6 hand surgery practices in the Netherlands at an average follow-up of 10 weeks (range, 6–12 weeks) after surgery. Using the Michigan Hand Outcomes Questionnaire, they determined that, compared with limited fasciectomy, patients who underwent NA had greater satisfaction, work performance, activities of daily living, and overall hand function. They had a similar rate of contracture correction (21° vs 18° total residual extension deficit) and a lower complication rate (5% vs 24%).

Quality-Adjusted Life Years, Costs

Chen and colleagues[21] studied the quality-adjusted life years (QALY) gained with Dupuytren treatment. The cost per QALY gained was $820,114 for an open partial fasciectomy; $49,995 or $166,268 for collagenase C histolyticum based on a collagenase market price of $945 or $5400 respectively; and $36,570 for NA when performed without a surgical center, anesthesiologist, or hand therapy. They concluded that open partial fasciectomy is not cost-effective.

Baltzer and Binhammer[67] developed an expected-value decision analysis model using health care and patient-incurred costs to compare open fasciotomy, NA, and collagenase. They also determined that fasciotomy was not cost-effective. NA was the most cost-effective treatment of single finger contractures, unless collagenase had a market price of $470 or less. Maravic and Beaudreuil[68] found that replacing open fasciectomy with NA could reduce treatments costs by 90% and overall health care costs by 56% to 59% for patients with Dupuytren with single-digit disease in France.

Plantar Fibromatosis

The authors have treated a small number of patients with plantar fibromatosis (Ledderhose disease) with NA. However, this treatment is less commonly indicated because flexion contractures are less frequent in the toes compared with the fingers. Plantar disease results in nodules more

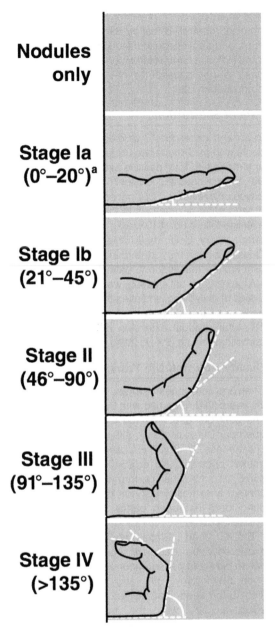

Nodules only

Stage Ia (0°–20°)[a]

Stage Ib (21°–45°)

Stage II (46°–90°)

Stage III (91°–135°)

Stage IV (>135°)

Fig. 6. Tubiana stage of Dupuytren's disease, based on the total passive extension digit, measured in degrees. [a] Degrees indicate total flexion contracture. (*Adapted from* Bainbridge C, Dahlin LB, Szczypa PP, et al. Current trends in the surgical management of Dupuytren's disease in Europe: an analysis of patient charts. Eur Orthop Traumatol 2012;3(1):35; with permission.)

commonly than cords; customized footwear and observation are most commonly advised.

SUMMARY

NA is an effective treatment of Dupuytren flexion contractures. Compared with other treatments, it is less expensive, results in lower complication rates, has higher patient satisfaction, and does not impair flexion postoperatively. It is convenient for patients and the surgeons; only 1 clinic visit is required, minimal dressings are required, only local anesthesia is required, and hand therapy is not needed. The authors recommend that all hand surgeons consider NA as a first-line treatment of symptomatic Dupuytren contractures of the MCP and IP joints with a palpable cord.

REFERENCES

1. Habash A, Rinker B. Dupuytren's disease involving the wrist. J Hand Surg Am 2007;32(3):352–4.
2. Eaton C. How common is Dupuytren disease? 2017. Available at: https://dupuytrens.org/common-dupuytren-disease/. Accessed April 28, 2017.
3. Gerber RA, Perry R, Thompson R, et al. Dupuytren's contracture: a retrospective database analysis to assess clinical management and costs in England. BMC Musculoskelet Disord 2011;12:73.
4. Lermusiaux J, Debeyre N. L'actualite rhumatologique 1979 presente aux praticien. Expansion Scientifique Francaise 1980.
5. Badois FJ, Lermusiaux JL, Massé C, et al. Non-surgical treatment of Dupuytren disease using needle fasciotomy. Rev Rhum Ed Fr 1993;60(11):808–13 [in French].
6. Lermusiaux JL, Lellouche H, Badois JF, et al. How should Dupuytren's contracture be managed in 1997? Rev Rhum Engl Ed 1997;64(12):775–6.
7. van Rijssen AL, Werker PM. Percutaneous needle fasciotomy in Dupuytren's disease. J Hand Surg Br 2006;31(5):498–501.
8. Lipman MD, Carstensen SE, Deal DN. Trends in the treatment of Dupuytren disease in the United States between 2007 and 2014. Hand (N Y) 2017;12(1):13–20.
9. Zhao JZ, Hadley S, Floyd E, et al. The impact of collagenase Clostridium histolyticum introduction on Dupuytren treatment patterns in the United States. J Hand Surg Am 2016;41(10):963–8.
10. Nydick JA, Olliff BW, Garcia MJ, et al. A comparison of percutaneous needle fasciotomy and collagenase injection for Dupuytren disease. J Hand Surg Am 2013;38(12):2377–80.
11. Cheung K, Walley KC, Rozental TD. Management of complications of Dupuytren contracture. Hand Clin 2015;31(2):345–54.
12. Skov ST, Bisgaard T, Søndergaard P, et al. Injectable collagenase versus percutaneous needle fasciotomy for Dupuytren contracture in proximal interphalangeal joints: a randomized controlled trial. J Hand Surg Am 2017;42(5):321–8.e3.

13. Pess GM, Pess RM, Pess RA. Results of needle apo-neurotomy for Dupuytren contracture in over 1,000 fingers. J Hand Surg Am 2012;37(4):651–6.

14. Molenkamp S, Schouten TAM, Broekstra DC, et al. Early postoperative results of percutaneous needle fasciotomy in 451 patients with Dupuytren disease. Plast Reconstr Surg 2017;139(6):1415–21.

15. Vlot M, Werker P. Effectiveness of percutaneous needle fasciotomy for second or higher recurrence in Dupuytren contracture. In: Werker P, Eaton J, Reichert C, et al, editors. Dupuytren disease and related diseases - the cutting edge, vol. 1. Switzerland: Springer International Publishing; 2017. p. 179–84.

16. Herrera FA, Benham P, Suliman A, et al. Cost comparison of open fasciectomy versus percuta-neous needle aponeurotomy for treatment of Du-puytren contracture. Ann Plast Surg 2013;70(4): 454–6.

17. van Rijssen AL, Gerbrandy FS, Ter Linden H, et al. A comparison of the direct outcomes of percuta-neous needle fasciotomy and limited fasciectomy for Dupuytren's disease: a 6-week follow-up study. J Hand Surg Am 2006;31(5):717–25.

18. Eaton C. Evidence-based medicine: Dupuytren contracture. Plast Reconstr Surg 2014;133(5): 1241–51.

19. Coleman S, Gilpin D, Tursi J, et al. Multiple concur-rent collagenase *Clostridium histolyticum* injections to Dupuytren's cords: an exploratory study. BMC Musculoskelet Disord 2012;13:61.

20. Coleman S, Gilpin D, Kaplan FT, et al. Efficacy and safety of concurrent collagenase *Clostridium histoly-ticum* injections for multiple Dupuytren contractures. J Hand Surg Am 2014;39(1):57–64.

21. Chen NC, Shauver MJ, Chung KC. Cost-effective-ness of open partial fasciectomy, needle aponeurot-omy, and collagenase injection for Dupuytren contracture. J Hand Surg Am 2011;36(11):1826–34.e32.

22. Lalonde D, Martin A. Tumescent local anesthesia for hand surgery: improved results, cost effectiveness, and wide-awake patient satisfaction. Arch Plast Surg 2014;41(4):312–6.

23. Dahlin LB, Bainbridge C, Szczypa PP, et al. Current trends in the surgical management of Dupuytren's disease in Europe: the surgeon's perspective. Eur Orthop Traumatol 2012;3(1):25–30.

24. Pess G. Tips and pearls for PNF and collagenase: a ten-year personal experience. In: Werker P, Eaton J, Reichert C, editors. Dupuytren disease and related diseases - the cutting edge, vol. 1. 1st edition. Switzerland: Springer International Publishing; 2017. p. 161–70.

25. Scherman P, Jenmalm P, Dahlin LB. One-year results of needle fasciotomy and collagenase injection in treatment of Dupuytren's contracture: a two-centre

26. Herrera FA, Mitchell S, Elzik M, et al. Modified percu-taneous needle aponeurotomy for the treatment of Dupuytren's contracture: early results and complica-tions. Hand (N Y) 2015;10(3):433–7.

27. Tosti R, Fowler J, Dwyer J, et al. Is antibiotic prophy-laxis necessary in elective soft tissue hand surgery? Orthopedics 2012;35(6):e829–33.

28. Bykowski MR, Sivak WN, Cray J, et al. Assessing the impact of antibiotic prophylaxis in outpatient elective hand surgery: a single-center, retrospective review of 8,850 cases. J Hand Surg Am 2011;36(11): 1741–7.

29. Dunn JC, Fares AB, Kusnezov N, et al. Current evi-dence regarding routine antibiotic prophylaxis in hand surgery. Hand (N Y) 2017;13(3):259–63.

30. Pereira C, Benhaim P. Needle aponeurotomy in the management of Dupuytren's contracture [Chapter 2]. In: Rizzo M, editor. Dupuytren's contracture, a clinical casebook. 1st edition. Switzerland: Springer; 2016. p. 13–37.

31. Donaldson J, Goddard N. The re-emergence of percutaneous fasciotomy in the management of Du-puytren's disease. Open Orthop J 2012;6:83–7.

32. Eaton C. A technique of needle aponeurotomy for Dupuytren's contracture. In: Eaton C, Seegenschmiedt M, Bayat A, et al, editors. Dupuytren's disease and related hyperproliferative disorders. Hei-delberg (Germany): Springer; 2012. p. 267–79.

33. Denkler KA, Vaughn CJ, Dolan EL, et al. Evidence-based medicine: options for Dupuytren's contrac-ture: incise, excise, and dissolve. Plast Reconstr Surg 2017;139(1):240e–55e.

34. Ketchum LD, Robinson DW, Masters FW. The degra-dation of mature collagen: a laboratory study. Plast Reconstr Surg 1967;40(1):89–91.

35. Ketchum LD, Donahue TK. The injection of nodules of Dupuytren's disease with triamcinolone aceto-nide. J Hand Surg Am 2000;25(6):1157–62.

36. McMillan C, Binhammer P. Steroid injection and nee-dle aponeurotomy for Dupuytren contracture: a ran-domized, controlled study. J Hand Surg Am 2012; 37(7):1307–12.

37. Hovius SE, Kan HJ, Smit X, et al. Extensive percuta-neous aponeurotomy and lipografting: a new treat-ment for Dupuytren disease. Plast Reconstr Surg 2011;128(1):221–8.

38. Kan HJ, Selles RW, van Nieuwenhoven CA, et al. Percutaneous aponeurotomy and lipofilling (PALF) versus limited fasciectomy in patients with primary Dupuytren's contracture: a prospective, random-ized, controlled trial. Plast Reconstr Surg 2016; 137(6):1800–12.

39. Sakellariou VI, Brault J, Rizzo M. Ultrasound-assis-ted percutaneous needle fasciotomy for Dupuytren's contracture. Orthopedics 2015;38(5):299–303.

prospective randomized clinical trial. J Hand Surg Eur Vol 2016;41(6):577–82.

40. Chen NC, Srinivasan RC, Shauver MJ, et al. A systematic review of outcomes of fasciotomy, aponeurotomy, and collagenase treatments for Dupuytren's contracture. Hand (N Y) 2011;6(3):250–5.

41. Denkler K. Surgical complications associated with fasciectomy for Dupuytren's disease: a 20-year review of the English literature. Eplasty 2010;10:e15.

42. Beaudreuil J, Lellouche H, Orcel P, et al. Needle aponeurotomy in Dupuytren's disease. Joint Bone Spine 2012;79(1):13–6.

43. Foucher G, Medina J, Navarro R. Percutaneous needle aponeurotomy: complications and results. J Hand Surg Br 2003;28(5):427–31.

44. Ullah AS, Dias JJ, Bhowal B. Does a 'firebreak' full-thickness skin graft prevent recurrence after surgery for Dupuytren's contracture?: a prospective, randomised trial. J Bone Joint Surg Br 2009;91(3):374–8.

45. Bulstrode NW, Jemec B, Smith PJ. The complications of Dupuytren's contracture surgery. J Hand Surg Am 2005;30(5):1021–5.

46. Spiers JD, Ullah A, Dias JJ. Vascular complication after collagenase injection and manipulation for Dupuytren's contracture. J Hand Surg Eur Vol 2014; 39(5):554–6.

47. Cheng HS, Hung LK, Tse WL, et al. Needle aponeurotomy for Dupuytren's contracture. J Orthop Surg (Hong Kong) 2008;16(1):88–90.

48. Swartz WM, Lalonde DH. MOC-PS(SM) CME article: Dupuytren's disease. Plast Reconstr Surg 2008; 121(4 Suppl):1–10.

49. Hurst LC, Badalamente MA, Hentz VR, et al. Injectable collagenase clostridium histolyticum for Dupuytren's contracture. N Engl J Med 2009;361(10): 968–79.

50. Crean SM, Gerber RA, Le Graverand MP, et al. The efficacy and safety of fasciectomy and fasciotomy for Dupuytren's contracture in European patients: a structured review of published studies. J Hand Surg Eur Vol 2011;36(5):396–407.

51. Hentz VR, Watt AJ, Desai SS, et al. Advances in the management of Dupuytren disease: collagenase. Hand Clin 2012;28(4):551–63.

52. Eaton C. Percutaneous fasciotomy for Dupuytren's contracture. J Hand Surg Am 2011;36(5):910–5.

53. Krauss EM, Lalonde DH. Secondary healing of fingertip amputations: a review. Hand (N Y) 2014; 9(3):282–8.

54. Smack DP, Harrington AC, Dunn C, et al. Infection and allergy incidence in ambulatory surgery patients using white petrolatum vs bacitracin ointment. A randomized controlled trial. JAMA 1996;276(12): 972–7.

55. Alqahtani M, Lalonde DH. Sterile versus nonsterile clean dressings. Can J Plast Surg 2006;14(1):25–7.

56. Grandizio LC, Akoon A, Heimbach J, et al. The use of residual collagenase for single digits with multiple-joint Dupuytren contractures. J Hand Surg Am 2017;42(6):472.e1-6.

57. Ebskov LB, Boeckstyns ME, Sørensen AI, et al. Results after surgery for severe Dupuytren's contracture: does a dynamic extension splint influence outcome? Scand J Plast Reconstr Surg Hand Surg 2000;34(2):155–60.

58. Jerosch-Herold C, Shepstone L, Chojnowski AJ, et al. Night-time splinting after fasciectomy or dermo-fasciectomy for Dupuytren's contracture: a pragmatic, multi-centre, randomised controlled trial. BMC Musculoskelet Disord 2011;12:136.

59. Pratt AL, Ball C. What are we measuring? A critique of range of motion methods currently in use for Dupuytren's disease and recommendations for practice. BMC Musculoskelet Disord 2016;17:20.

60. Rahr L, Søndergaard P, Bisgaard T, et al. Percutaneous needle fasciotomy for primary Dupuytren's contracture. J Hand Surg Eur Vol 2011;36(7): 548–52.

61. Hindocha S, Stanley JK, Watson S, et al. Dupuytren's diathesis revisited: evaluation of prognostic indicators for risk of disease recurrence. J Hand Surg Am 2006;31(10):1626–34.

62. van Rijssen AL, ter Linden H, Werker PM. Five-year results of a randomized clinical trial on treatment in Dupuytren's disease: percutaneous needle fasciotomy versus limited fasciectomy. Plast Reconstr Surg 2012;129(2):469–77.

63. Peimer CA, Blazar P, Coleman S, et al. Dupuytren contracture recurrence following treatment with collagenase Clostridium histolyticum (CORDLESS study): 3-year data. J Hand Surg Am 2013;38(1): 12–22.

64. Strömberg J, Ibsen-Sörensen A, Fridén J. Comparison of treatment outcome after collagenase and needle fasciotomy for Dupuytren contracture: a randomized, single-blinded, clinical trial with a 1-year follow-up. J Hand Surg Am 2016;41(9):873–80.

65. Zhou C, Selles RW, Slijper HP, et al. Comparative effectiveness of percutaneous needle aponeurotomy and limited fasciectomy for Dupuytren's contracture: a multicenter observational study. Plast Reconstr Surg 2016;138(4):837–46.

66. Bainbridge C, Dahlin LB, Szczypa PP, et al. Current trends in the surgical management of Dupuytren's disease in Europe: an analysis of patient charts. Eur Orthop Traumatol 2012;3(1):31–41.

67. Baltzer H, Binhammer PA. Cost-effectiveness in the management of Dupuytren's contracture. A Canadian cost-utility analysis of current and future management strategies. Bone Joint J 2013;95-B(8): 1094–100.

68. Maravic M, Beaudreuil J. Impact on costs of switching one-ray aponeurectomy to percutaneous needle aponeurotomy in Dupuytren's disease: a model analysis. Joint Bone Spine 2015;82(4):264–6.

Development of Collagenase Treatment for Dupuytren Disease

Marie A. Badalamente, PhD[a],*, Lawrence C. Hurst, MD[b]

KEYWORDS

- Dupuytren disease • Collagenase *Clostridium histolyticum* (CCH) injection • CCH development
- Treatment

KEY POINTS

- Collagenase *Clostridium histolyticum* (CCH) injection was first developed in laboratory study before human clinical trials.
- US Food and Drug Administration (FDA)-regulated phase 2 single-center and multicenter clinical trials defined the CCH injection method targeting the Dupuytren cord and the minimum safe and effective dose.
- US FDA-regulated phase 3 multicenter trials in the United States and Australia showed CCH injection was safe and effective.

Collagenase is a well-known and studied enzyme. Ines Mandl,[1] from the Polytechnic Institute of Brooklyn, studied, isolated, and characterized collagenase from *Clostridium histolyticum* in 1953.

Drs Badalamente and Hurst[2–4] had performed many basic-science studies on Dupuytren disease, and by the early 1990s became interested in targeting the collagen cord as a means of therapeutic treatment. Collagenase came to mind, but many obstacles were present. First, the concern for normal collagen-containing structures of the human finger was paramount. Second, there was no animal model of the disorder. Finally, the funding and time necessary for such translational, "bench-to-bedside" research would be enormous.

PRECLINICAL STUDIES

Our studies began in a rat-tail animal model,[5] which we chose for the structural similarity to a human finger, as collagenous structures of the tendons are in close proximity to neurovascular structures and bone. Using this model, the right sacrocaudalis ventralis lateralis (tail) tendon was surgically exposed in adult male rats and injected with purified collagenase *Clostridium histolyticum* (CCH) (0.054 mg in 10 μL neutral buffer or 0.108 mg in 10 μL buffer, n = 7 per group) or a control solution (10 μL of sterile buffer, n = 7). In each group, 4 animals were euthanized at 1 hour postinjection, and 4 animals were euthanized at 24 hours postinjection. A 2-cm portion of each tail (including the injection site) was prepared for histologic analysis.

Tissue prepared from control animals showed intact collagen bundles and adjacent skin. At all doses used, collagen lysis of the injected tendons was apparent. Most importantly, in all animals receiving collagenase, no extravasation of collagenase to adjacent tissues was noted, and no

Disclosures: The authors are consultants for Endo Pharmaceuticals, Ashai-Kasei Pharmaceuticals and receive partial Xiaflex/Xiapex royalties from Biospecifics Technologies Corp.
a Department of Orthopaedics, T-18 Health Science Center, Stony Brook University Medical Center, Room 052, 100 Nicolls Road, Stony Brook, NY 11794, USA; b Department of Orthopaedics, T-18 Health Science Center, Stony Brook University Medical Center, Room 080, Stony Brook, NY 11794, USA
* Corresponding author.
E-mail address: Marie.Badalamente@stonybrookmedicine.edu

Hand Clin 34 (2018) 345–349
https://doi.org/10.1016/j.hcl.2018.03.004
0749-0712/18/© 2018 Elsevier Inc. All rights reserved.

micro-hemorrhage other than that associated with the surgical procedure was present. All adjacent structures, including ventral artery and vein, nerve bundles, muscle, and skin, remained intact and showed normal anatomy (**Fig. 1**). Tissue proximal and distal to the injection site also showed normal anatomy.

Laboratory bench study[6] continued using 20 Dupuytren cords, which were surgically removed from patients at fasciectomy and randomly assigned to treatment with collagenase injection (0.054 mg, 0.108 mg, or 0.216 mg) or control buffer injection. Twenty-four hours after treatment, mechanical testing of tensile modulus was performed, during which cords were placed under a constant displacement of 9 mm/s until cord rupture. This study showed a clear inverse relationship between collagenase dose and decreasing stress. Comparison of these data with previous reports of the average muscle tendon extensor force of each finger suggested that 0.108 mg collagenase was the minimum effective dose sufficient to cause cord rupture by the normal extensor forces of the index, long, ring, and small fingers. Furthermore, histologic examination of collagenase-treated cords revealed collagen lysis, which was increasingly apparent with incremental doses of collagenase.

FIRST CLINICAL STUDY

It was now time to approach the US Food and Drug Administration (FDA) on 2 fronts. The first was to secure an Investigational New Drug (IND) number, which would allow for human clinical studies, with Drs Badalamente and Hurst as sponsor/investigators of the IND, which did not involve industry support. The second was to submit a grant proposal to the FDA for funding of the

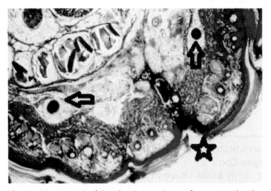

Fig. 1. Transverse histologic section of a rat tail. The collagenase injection track is shown at the star. The arrows denote normal tendons. The tendon within the collagenase injection track has been lysed by the enzyme.

clinical studies. In the mid-1990s, the IND was granted, and we were successful in obtaining the FDA funding.

We relied first on the laboratory biomechanical results, which indicated that 0.054 mg injectable collagenase would be sufficient to lyse a cord in a patient with Dupuytren disease. The injection in the first patient at this dose was safe, but did not induce cord rupture. With FDA guidance and permission, we increased the injectable collagenase dosages in the next 5 patients, which was safe, but again did not elicit cord rupture. Disheartened, and on the brink of abandoning the work, we decided to administer 0.58 mg injectable collagenase to a patient with a 30° contracture of the ring finger. At 24 hours postinjection, we gently manipulated the finger in extension, heard a "cracking" sound, and saw that the cord had been safely and completely ruptured. The patient was able to flex and extend the finger immediately and normally. Adverse events, which we now know to be quite common after this procedure, were seen in this first successfully treated patient. They were pain at the injection area, edema, and bruising, which abated in 7 to 14 days.

The remaining 29 patients in this first clinical study[7] received injections of 0.58 mg collagenase. Repeat injections were given 4 to 6 weeks apart if the joint angle did not correct to within 0° to 5°. Thirty of 34 metacarpophalangeal (MP) joints (88%) and 4 of 9 proximal interphalangeal (PIP) joints (44%) treated with 0.58 mg collagenase were fully corrected to 0° extension, or improved to within 5° extension. An average of 1 injection was required to achieve these results.

PHASE 2 STUDIES

A single-center, randomized, placebo-controlled, double-blind, phase 2a study[8] was subsequently conducted in 49 patients: 36 patients with MP joint contracture and 13 patients with PIP joint contracture. The primary efficacy endpoint was correction of contracture to within 0° to 5° of normal extension (0°) within 30 days of the last injection. Patients not meeting the primary endpoint after 1 injection in the double-blind study could receive up to 4 additional injections of 0.58 mg of collagenase on an optional, open-label basis. The open-label extension was available to all patients, including those randomized to receive placebo during the double-blind phase. One month after injection with collagenase, 14 (78%) of 18 MP joints showed correction of contracture to within 0° to 5° extension compared with 2 (11%) of 18 MP joints after injection with placebo. The 4 patients who did not achieve correction of deformity to within

0° to 5° with the first injection of collagenase were treated again, and all showed correction of contracture to within 0° to 5° 1 month after the second injection. Of the patients with PIP joint contractures, 5 (71%) of 7 treated with collagenase and none treated with placebo were corrected to 0° to 5° 1 month postinjection. Flexion and grip strength did not significantly change compared with baseline values.

An important aspect of this early phase 2a study was to monitor adverse events and any potential adverse immune reactions. As with the first patient successfully treated, pain in the injection area, edema, and bruising occurred and resolved within 7 to 14 days. Antibody assays for anti-collagenase immunoglobulin (Ig)G and IgE were elevated, but no adverse effects were detected in patients.

In the next phase 2b study,[9,10] the FDA asked us to consider if, indeed, 0.58 mg of injectable collagenase was the minimum safe and effective dose. We enlisted the help of our friend and colleague, Dr Vincent R. Hentz, at Stanford University. Subsequently, 80 patients took part in a randomized, double-blind, placebo-controlled, dose-response, phase 2b trial conducted at Stony Brook University Medical Center and Stanford University.

Fifty-five patients had MP joint contractures and 25 had PIP joint contractures. Joints were randomized to receive a single injection of 0.145 mg, 0.29 mg, or 0.58 mg collagenase or placebo. A comparison of dose groups showed that in both MP and PIP joints, the return to normal extension (0° to 5°) was higher in patients who received 0.58 mg of collagenase 1 month after injection compared with the lower collagenase doses or placebo. Of the patients receiving 0.58 mg of collagenase, 78% achieved normal extension by 1 month. In comparison, the 0.29-mg and 0.145-mg dose groups achieved normal extension in 45% and 50% of patients, respectively. No response was observed in the placebo group. An open-label extension of this study permitted up to 4 additional 0.58-mg collagenase injections. Adverse events were similar to the phase 2a study.

INITIAL PHASE 3 STUDY

At the end of phase 2, a meeting was then held with the FDA, after which permission was given to proceed to phase 3 studies. At this point in time, it was a disappointment to Drs Badalamente and Hurst that no industry sponsors would consider funding the work. Therefore, we decided to advance to phase 3 study at our own institution, with the continued FDA funding.

A single-center phase 3 trial at our institution, Stony Brook University Medical Center (Stony Brook, Long Island, NY) was then conducted. This study included 35 patients who were randomized in a 2:1 ratio to receive injections of collagenase (n = 23; 0.58 mg) or placebo (n = 12). Primary and, when possible, secondary and tertiary joints were identified for each patient, resulting in a total of 55 affected joints. Patients could receive up to 3 injections in the primary joint 4 to 6 weeks apart. Those who achieved correction to 0° to 5° extension after the first injection were eligible to be re-randomized to further treatment for a secondary or tertiary joint. All patients wore splints at night for 4 months after injection. The primary efficacy endpoint was a reduction in deformity in the primary joint to within 0° to 5° 30 days after the last injection. Additional endpoints included time to clinical success, number of injections required to achieve correction to 0° to 5° of normal, and recurrence (defined as return of contracture ≥20° in successfully treated joints).

Of the 35 randomized patients, 33 completed the double-blind study. In addition, 9 patients were re-randomized after successful treatment of the primary joint: 6 received collagenase, and 3 received placebo. One tertiary joint was also treated with collagenase. Overall, 21 (91%) of 23 patients who received collagenase and 0 (0%) of 12 who received placebo for a primary joint achieved 0° to 5° extension. Both joint types responded well to collagenase treatment with correction to 0° to 5° attained in 12 (86%) of 14 MP joints, and 9 (100%) of 9 PIP joints (**Figs. 2 and 3**). Furthermore, 16 of 23 patients achieved correction to 0° to 5° with a single collagenase injection, whereas 2 patients required 2 injections, and 3 patients required 3 injections.

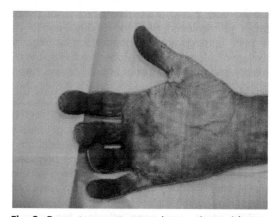

Fig. 2. Dupuytren contracture in a patient with contractures of the index, long, ring, and little finger PIP joints.

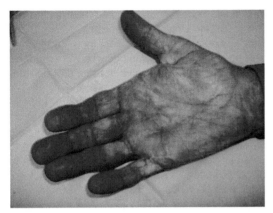

Fig. 3. The same patient as shown in **Fig. 2** after collagenase injections to his PIP joints, showing improved extension.

Overall, for the primary joint treated, the mean number of injections for correction to 0° to 5° was 1.4, and median time to clinical success was 8 days. Correction to 0° to 5° was also achieved in 5 (83%) of 6 collagenase-treated secondary joints, and in the one collagenase-treated tertiary joint.

Patients in the double-blind phase 3 study who failed to achieve correction to 0° to 5°, or who had other involved joints of the same or contralateral hand, were eligible to continue treatment in the open-label extension study.

ADVERSE EVENTS

In general, collagenase therapy was well tolerated in phase 2 and phase 3 clinical studies, with all adverse events graded as mild to moderate, and most resolving within approximately 1 to 3 weeks. Injection-site pain, hand ecchymosis, and edema were the most frequently reported adverse events in both double-blind and open-label phase 2 and phase 3 studies, with mean times to resolution of 8 to 15 days and 2 to 9 days, respectively. Lymphadenopathy (usually axillary or elbow) was also observed in approximately one-third of patients in both phase 2 and phase 3 studies.

There were 11 skin lacerations at the time of cord rupture in the phase 3 studies (3 in the double-blind study and 8 in the open-label study) and 3 in the phase 2 studies, with none occurring in placebo patients. These lacerations occurred primarily in patients who had experienced severe (>80°) baseline contracture over many years. All lacerations were effectively healed through secondary intent, and none affected the clinical outcome. Finally, no systemic immunologic adverse events were reported.

INDUSTRY SPONSORSHIP

Pivotal phase 3 study still needed to be performed and funded before data could be submitted to the FDA in a Biologics License Application for a new drug approval. Fortunately, an industry sponsor was identified in Auxilium Pharmaceuticals in Malvern, PA. Our FDA IND number was therefore transferred to Auxilium, and multicenter phase 3 trials at 15 sites in the United States (CORD 1) and 5 sites in Australia (CORD 2) commenced. It had been approximately 12 years from the publication of the first laboratory "bench" studies to the point in time when we began the pivotal phase 3 studies.

In the CORD studies,[11] more than 300 patients were enrolled and were required to have a minimum 20° contracture. They were randomized using a ratio of 2:1 to receive collagenase (0.58 mg) or placebo. The primary objective of CORD 1 and CORD 2 was correction of the joint contracture to within 0° to 5° after up to 3 injections of study treatment. On completion of a double-blind phase, patients who initially received placebo or who had other affected joints were eligible for enrollment in open-label extension phases during which all patients received 0.58-mg collagenase treatment.

Overall, 64% of joints treated with collagenase versus 6.8% treated with placebo were corrected to 0° to 5° after the last injection in CORD 1. In CORD 2, the rates were 44.4% versus 4.8%, respectively. The most common adverse events reported in CORD 1 and 2 were pain, swelling, bruising, and pruritus at the injection site. No systemic allergic reactions were reported. Overall, 7 serious adverse events possibly related to

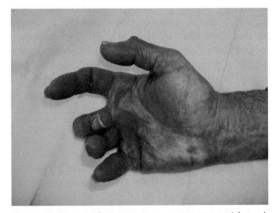

Fig. 4. Patient with Dupuytren contracture with multiple contractures of MP and PIP joints of the index, long, ring, and little fingers. This was recurrent after surgical fasciectomy. The patient was treated using 2 (0.58-mg) collagenase doses.

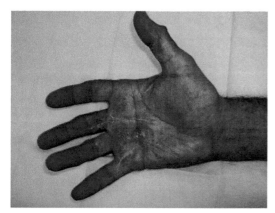

Fig. 5. The same patient as shown in **Fig. 4** 30 days after treatment showing a very good/excellent result for each finger treated.

collagenase were reported: 2 confirmed tendon ruptures, 1 pulley ligament injury, and 1 complex regional pain syndrome.

In September 2009, an FDA Advisory Committee met to review all the data and voted 12 to 0 for approval of collagenase injection(s) in adult patients with Dupuytren disease with a palpable cord. The drug is marketed as Xiaflex in the United States. Subsequently, regulatory agencies around the world, including the European Union (Xiapex), Swiss Medic, Health Canada, the Australian Therapeutic Goods Administration, and the Japanese Regulatory Agency also approved collagenase injection. In October 2014, concurrent use of 2 (0.58-mg) doses in the same hand, with or without delayed finger manipulation, was approved by the FDA to address treatment of multiple contractures (**Figs. 4** and **5**). In January 2015, Endo Pharmaceuticals completed the acquisition of Auxilium Pharmaceuticals and now markets the drug.

REFERENCES

1. Mandl I, MacLennan JD, Howes EL, et al. Isolation and characterization of proteinase and collagenase from *Clostridium histolyticum*. J Clin Invest 1953; 32(12):1323–9.
2. Badalamente MA, Hurst LC, Sampson SP. Prostaglandins influence myofibroblast contractility in Dupuytren's disease. J Hand Surg 1988;13A(6): 867–71.
3. Badalamente MA, Hurst LC, Grandia S, et al. Platelet derived growth factor in Dupuytren's disease. J Hand Surg 1992;17(A):317–23.
4. Badalamente MA, Sampson SP, Hurst LC, et al. The role of transforming growth factor beta in Dupuytren's disease. J Hand Surg 1996;21A:210–5.
5. Badalamente MA, Hurst LC. Enzyme injection as a nonoperative treatment for Dupuytren's disease. Drug Deliv 1996;3(1):35–40.
6. Starkweather K, Lattuga S, Hurst LC, et al. Collagenase in the treatment of Dupuytren's disease: an in vitro study. J Hand Surg 1996;21A:490–5.
7. Hurst LC, Badalamente MA. Nonoperative treatment of Dupuytren's disease. In: Rayan GM, editor. Hand clinics. Philadelphia: WB Saunders; 1999. p. 97–107.
8. Badalamente MA, Hurst LC. Enzyme injection as a nonoperative treatment of Dupuytren's disease. J Hand Surg 2000;25A(4):629–36.
9. Badalamente MA, Hurst LC, Hentz VR. Collagen as a clinical target: nonoperative treatment of Dupuytren's disease. J Hand Surg 2002;27A(5):788–98.
10. Badalamente MA, Hurst LC. Efficacy and safety of injectable mixed collagenase subtypes in the treatment of Dupuytren's contracture. J Hand Surg 2007;32(6):767–74.
11. Hurst LC, Badalamente MA, Hentz VR, et al. Injectable collagenase *Clostridium histolyticum* for Dupuytren's contracture. N Engl J Med 2009;361: 968–79.

Fasciectomy for Dupuytren Contracture

Joseph J. Dias, MBBS, FRCS (Eng), MD (Res)*, Sheweidin Aziz, MBBS, MRCS (Eng)

KEYWORDS

- Dupuytren • Fasciectomy • Surgery • Complications

KEY POINTS

- Know the anatomy of Dupuytren's cords causing contracture. Be aware of the spiral nerve.
- The role of minimal goal surgery should be understood and the procedure stopped once adequate correction is achieved without persevering to get full correction.
- For a stiff PIP joint sequential releases are done step-by-step. At each step formally decide whether to proceed or accept the correction achieved.
- Small wounds of up to 1.5 cm may be left open in the digits; larger wounds may be left open in the palm to heal by secondary intention.
- Early rehabilitation and encouragement of independence with activities of daily living is highly recommended.

INTRODUCTION

Dupuytren disease, or palmar fibromatosis, is a benign yet disabling, irreversible, progressive fibroproliferative condition affecting the palm and fingers, leading to flexion contractures of the metacarpophalangeal (MCP) and proximal interphalangeal (PIP) joints.

Worldwide, 4% to 6% of caucasians are affected by Dupuytren disease.[1] Increasing age and male gender are linked to a higher incidence and severity of the disease.[2] Other risk factors include diabetes mellitus, epilepsy, manual labor, alcoholism, and smoking.[3–5] Family history and genetic predisposition have been linked to Dupuytren disease.[6] The progressive extension deficit encroaches on the working space of the hand.

INDICATIONS: WHEN TO CONSIDER SURGERY

Dupuytren disease is usually a painless condition, although patients may complain of pain when gripping due to the pressure exerted over the nodules in the palm. Patients initially present with skin pits, nodules, or distortion of palmar creases, which may develop into cords, and these can cause joint contracture. Dimples are caused by thickening and tethering of the vertical fascial fibers to the dermis.[1]

Usually the primary complaint is progressive bending of a digit associated with a cord or nodule; this may affect a patient's daily living activities. The Hueston tabletop test[7] is positive if a patient is unable to place a hand flat on the table, and this usually reflects a contracture of more than 30° at the MCP joint and/or the PIP joint. This provides the threshold where clinicians may consider treatment.

The aim of intervention is to regain extension of the affected joint(s) and improve function.

Factors influencing management decisions include

1. Disease factors: contracture location, severity, and diathesis
2. Patient factors: general condition, comorbidity, and anesthetic risk

AToMS-Academic Team of Musculoskeletal Surgery, Undercroft, University Hospitals of Leicester NHS Trust, Leicester General Hospital, Gwendolen Road, Leicester, LE5 4PW, UK
* Corresponding author.
E-mail address: jd96@leicester.ac.uk

Hand Clin 34 (2018) 351–366
https://doi.org/10.1016/j.hcl.2018.04.002

3. Surgeon factors: skill, repertoire, and expertise
4. Availability of postoperative care and occupational/hand therapy to recover hand function

Dupuytren diathesis constitutes a group of characteristics that predispose those affected to a more severe form of Dupuytren disease and increased risk of recurrence. An assessment of diathesis helps choose a treatment option and advise the patient on the likelihood of recurrence. First described by Hueston[8] in 1963, these characteristics include

1. Bilateral disease
2. Positive family history with focus on first-degree and second-degree relatives
3. Presence of ectopic disease
   a. Ledderhose disease—plantar fibromatosis
   b. Peyronie disease—induration and deformity of the penis
   c. Garrod knuckle pads—nodular thickenings over the dorsum of the PIP joints
4. Young age of onset (before 45 years)[9]

These characteristics suggest a more severe phenotype of the disease. Histologic analysis of skin and underlying cord may identify fibroblasts positive for smooth muscle α-actin within the dermis, and this, too, is associated with higher recurrence rates.[10] It is, however, unusual to request this investigation.

Other factors that need to be considered include

1. The total number of digits affected
2. The total number of surgical procedures performed, because this identifies the high risk of recurrence

Preoperative measurement of contractures at MCP and PIP joints should be recorded using a goniometer with wrist in a neutral position to exclude the fasciodesis effect. Identification of the fasciodesis effect—where the joint contracture angle changes when the position of the wrist or MCP joint is changed—is a sign that good correction is likely after surgery.

The severity of Dupuytren contracture is commonly determined using the Tubiana staging system[11]; it accounts for total flexion deformity in joints of a single affected digit (**Table 1**). Total flexion deformity is calculated as the angle between the dorsum of the hand and the middle phalanx. Tubiana and colleagues does not distinguish between MCP and PIP disease.[12]

In addition to the contracture, the authors also note the site and size of nodules and cords, the

Table 1	
Tubiana staging for Dupuytren contracture	
Stage	**Deformity**
0	No lesion
N	Palmar nodule without presence of contracture
1	Contracture between 0° and 45°
2	Contracture between 45° and 90°
3	Contracture between 90° and 135°
4	Contracture >135°

Adapted from Hindocha S, Stanley JK, Watson JS, et al. Revised Tubiana's staging system for assessment of disease severity in Dupuytren's disease-preliminary clinical findings. Hand 2008;3(2):81; with permission.

type of skin (whether it is thick and calloused or supple and mobile), and whether it is tethered or mobile over the cord(s). The authors record the flexion range at each joint (**Fig. 1**).

ANATOMY OF DUPUYTREN DISEASE

A good understanding of the anatomy of the fascia is essential for safe and effective surgery.

The pathologic anatomy[13] is determined by the known anatomy of the fascia of the palm and fingers. Depending on which fascial structures become involved, cords may be central, spiral, or lateral. Knowledge of the fascial anatomy ensures safe and quick dissection of the cords causing contracture.

Grayson and Cleland ligaments hold the skin in position during flexion and extension of the finger. Cleland ligaments are firm fascia cords that run from the side of the phalanges to the skin, dorsal to the neurovascular bundles. Cleland ligaments were previously believed not involved in Dupuytren disease; however, they do contribute to PIP joint contracture.[14]

The natatory ligament, otherwise known as superficial transverse metacarpal ligament, are ligamentous fibers that extend between metacarpals in the web spaces of the digits and lie immediately beneath the skin and help create the web space. Digital nerves and vessels pass deep and dorsal to the natatory ligament. It tightens as the digit abducts. In Dupuytren disease, there is thickening and contracture of the natatory ligament, or a cord arising from it, which leads to loss of abduction and decrease in finger span. Because the natatory ligament may coalesce with the lateral cord, this may also contribute to PIP joint contracture.

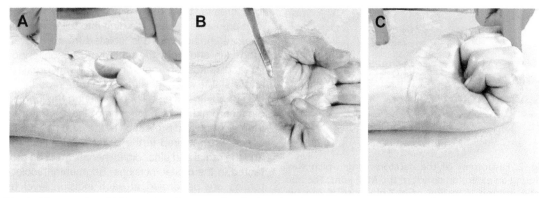

Fig. 1. (*A*) Lateral and (*B*) anterior photographs of a hand with Dupuytren contracture affecting the small finger of the left hand demonstrating severe contracture of the MCP and PIP joints. (*C*) The flexion photograph demonstrates full flexion is present before surgery.

SURGICAL OPTIONS

When the decision to offer treatment has been made, the surgeon should discuss the benefits and risks associated with each treatment option with the patient. Although patient wishes should be taken into account, the surgeon must decide whether a particular treatment is likely to improve function. This discussion should be documented in a patient's chart. Generally, patients should be operated on as soon as possible to avoid worsening of contracture. The authors obtain consent prior to the day of surgery to give patients ample time to consider the information.

The procedures are performed as day case surgery under general, regional, or local anesthesia. If not used during the case, local anesthetic (eg, levobupivacaine or bupivacaine) infiltration at the end of surgery as ring and/or ulnar nerve block can improve postoperative pain control.

Surgical intervention for Dupuytren contractures achieves a high rate of full or almost full correction (75%). Surgery may also be associated with a high rate of patient-reported postoperative complications (46%), but most are minor and resolve over time without specific intervention. The rate of surgical complications, persistence, and recurrence is higher in patients with worse initial deformities.[15]

In the operating theater, the patient is positioned supine with the arm abducted on an arm table.

A wide pneumatic tourniquet cuff is carefully applied with at least 3 layers of cast padding applied between tourniquet and skin, making sure there is an overlap of padding at the edge of the tourniquet. The self-regulated pneumatic tourniquet set at approximately 250 mm Hg (may be higher or lower according to body habitus and systolic blood pressure) aids in visualization of the neurovascular structures. The arm is elevated just before inflating the tourniquet; the authors do not use a bandage to exsanguinate the arm. The use of loupes to magnify the view facilitates identification of neurovascular structures because Dupuytren disease can distort normal anatomy.

FASCIOTOMY

Open fasciotomy may be performed for some bands or as minimal goals surgery if patients are not fit for regional or general anesthesia. Minimal goals surgery may be due to age, multiple comorbidities, or patient preference to avoid wider surgery. Minimal goals surgery is where patient and surgeon agree that the objective is to improve the extension deficit but both wish to avoid extensive surgery with its greater risk and longer recovery. This often means focusing on isolated, high-yield joint releases without pursuing aggressive surgery on other, less favorable joints. Minimal goals surgery may be considered in 3 situations: (1) in very comorbid patients, mainly because of anesthetic risks; (2) in the elderly because of frailty; and (3) in a long-standing contracture, where there is uncertainty as to the degree of correction that can be obtained.

This procedure can also be used after failed percutaneous needle fasciotomy or in more severe Dupuytren disease where visualization of the cord(s) is needed or cords are very thick. It is mainly used for MCP joint contractures (pretendinous cord) or for a symptomatic natatory cord. A small incision is made to visualize the cord/nodule and identify and preserve the neurovascular structures (**Fig. 2**). Once the cord is identified, it is then divided. The wound may or may not be closed primarily. Patients are able to return to their activities almost immediately after the procedure.

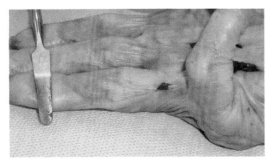

Fig. 2. Fasciotomy of the natatory cord, which was causing an extension deficit of the MCP joint. The oblique incision is in line of a Z-plasty so it can be extended if needed. The cord is identified, dissected, and divided. The wound can be left open if required.

FASCIECTOMY

Fasciectomy involves the removal of abnormal fascia to permit contracture correction. Targeted cord and nodules are excised from the affected digit(s) until correction is achieved. There are 2 recognized approaches to performing a fasciectomy; both have similar outcomes.

Segmental Fasciectomy

Described by Moermans in 1991,[16] the segmental fasciectomy technique uses C-shaped incisions (**Fig. 3**) of approximately 1-cm limbs. Alternatively, a series of transverse incisions of approximately 1 cm to 1.5 cm may be used, beginning over the distal palmar crease before proceeding distally as necessary in a stepwise fashion to the MCP

joint crease, the proximal phalanx, and the PIP joint crease to release the digit into full extension. The pretendinous cord is isolated from the overlying skin and from the underlying flexor tendon for a distance of approximately 1 cm proximal and distal to each incision. Localization and division of any transverse fibers tethering the longitudinal cord aid in the correction of the contracture. Identification and protection of the common digital nerves are required in the distal palmar incision, and the radial and ulnar digital nerves must be protected in the digital incisions. Segmental fasciectomies are performed at each incision level by taking out a section of the cord, leaving intermediate sections of diseased fascia undisturbed.[17]

Limited Fasciectomy

More commonly performed is limited fasciectomy described by Hueston[18] as excision of the palpably thickened fascia. This is described in step-by-step detail later.

DERMOFASCIECTOMY

Dermofasciectomy is a more extensive than limited fasciectomy procedure[19] used in patients with severe or recurrent Dupuytren disease. It has been described as a "preaxial amputation" of the digit, removing all tissue that may result in flexion contracture. It is performed using an oblique incision starting from the distal interphalangeal joint to the distal flexure palmar crease followed by a transverse palmar incision to make

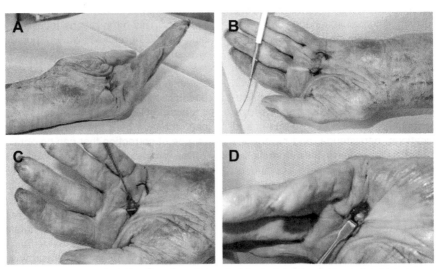

Fig. 3. Segmental fasciectomy is performed through small C-shaped incisions, through which short segments of Dupuytren cord can be excised at intervals. These small incisions may be very useful in elderly patients with very fragile skin. Wounds are gently closed, or may be left partly open if there is undue tension. (*A*) Multiple MCP deformity. (*B*) Segmental incisions. (*C, D*) Bands identified.

an L-type incision. The skin and the underlying abnormal fascia are removed as a single unit.

For wound coverage, a full-thickness skin graft may be harvested from the hypothenar region or the medial arm to cover the defect. A split-thickness skin graft is not used, because it is contracts more during healing. Full-thickness skin grafts on a well-vascularized bed can heal over a central avascular defect of up to 1 cm in diameter. These supple grafts can allow excellent recovery of flexion.[20]

LIMITED FASCIECTOMY SURGICAL PROCEDURE: TECHNIQUE
Step 1: Incision

Incisions are made to facilitate exposure and aid closure without tissue tension. Superficial identification of the Dupuytren cords and/or nodules and inspection of the overlying skin is done to decide on the best incision to perform the surgery as well as a tension-free wound closure. Skin is marked with a pen. The planned incision is made, and the skin is mobilized to expose the cord/nodule.

Incisions may be any of the following:

- Transverse: this may be used in open fasciotomy mainly in the palm, because it aids visualization of the affected cord as well as the neurovascular structures. This incision provides fast healing but may be difficult to close. It also allows cords to multiple digits to be addressed.
- Z-plasty: this is commonly used in Dupuytren disease, where skin closure may not be easily achieved (**Fig. 4**). Skoog[21] described a transverse incision in the palm extended via a longitudinal midline incision into the digit with Z-plasties made in the digit at the end of the procedure.
- Bruner (zig-zag): this may be used in mild to moderate Dupuytren disease, where the skin is likely to close with minimal tension and gap. It is an extensible approach and may be reused in future for revisions but permits only minimal lengthening. The authors rarely use this incision.
- Midlateral approach: this allows the bands predominantly on 1 side of the digit to be explored. It is easy to identify and protect the neurovascular bundles by approaching them through the Cleland fascia (**Fig. 5**).

The authors' preferred incision for complex Dupuytren disease is longitudinal, because it can be extended with Z-plasties. A single Z-plasty over the proximal phalanx is planned; the Z-plasty

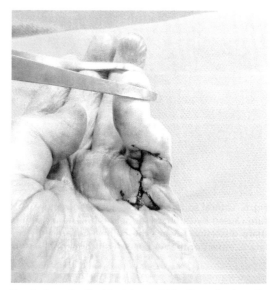

Fig. 4. Longitudinal incision, which allows for lengthening with Z-plasties. Two Z-plasties are typically made: 1 over the proximal phalanx and the other over the palm. The position of the flaps is based on where skin lengthening is required, while avoiding any element of the Z-plasty extending into the interspaces between the fingers where the perforators come from the dorsum to the superficial skin.

has a proximal flap on the more adherent side of the disease because this helps preserve the circulation into the apex. For the little finger, this usually is the ulnar flap as identification and release of the contracture cords arising from the abductor digiti minimi and inserting into the Cleland fascia at the middle phalanx is required. Often 2 Z-plasties that are made: 1 over the proximal phalanx and a second in the palm. The authors avoid incising the skin in the fatty interspace between the fingers, where the vascular perforator preserves circulation to the skin.

The skin is raised wherever the skin is mobile first. Fine skin hooks are used to provide tension to take down the adherent segments of the skin, which usually occurs over the PIP joint and over the proximal finger crease.

Step 2: Dissection of Diseased Fascia

Once the skin is raised, the principal cord is identified, and all extensions from the cord to the skin are divided (**Fig. 6**). Dissection deep to the transverse fascia in the palm is not required; however, the longitudinal cords that attach to the side of the A1 and A2 pulleys near the transverse fascia are divided. The transverse fascia is kept intact, protecting the neurovascular structures that lie deep to it.

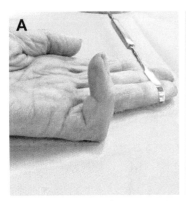
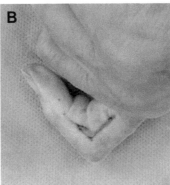
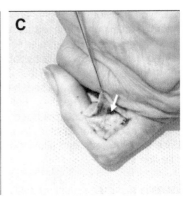

Fig. 5. Lateral approach to a PIP joint contracture. (*A*) Lateral view of the hand showing a severe PIP joint contracture caused by Dupuytren disease. (*B*) The incision is made in the midlateral line, and the flap mobilized with sharp dissection toward the palmar surface. (*C*) This shows the stout cord (*arrow*) from the MCP joint to the lateral aspect of the A4 pulley. Full correction was achieved after its excision.

The fascia should then be carefully dissected, dividing all the attachments to skin, and attention paid to finding the cord's distal insertion into the side of the A4 pulley. Sometimes, the cord can split in 2, wrapping around the A4 pulley (**Fig. 7**).

When dissecting at the level of the proximal phalanx, especially its proximal part, the authors watch carefully for fatty structures. When present, these are not divided until the neurovascular structures are identified, because within these tissues, the rare occurrence of a nerve spiraling the cord

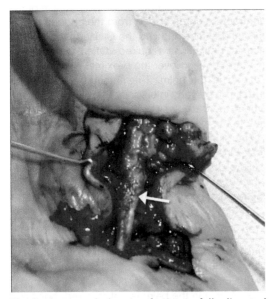

Fig. 6. Photograph showing fascia carefully dissected with all the bands that go to skin divided and the insertion of the cord onto the side of the A4 pulley (*arrow*). Note that the cord is not divided yet, because the tension in the cord can help facilitate the dissection.

might be found. The authors identify the nerve in front of the Cleland ligament and behind the Grayson ligament at the PIP joint and follow it proximally to ensure identification of a nerve, which spirals the cord.[22]

The neurovascular structures are dissected on their lateral side rather than their medial side to avoid damaging branches from the vessels and nerve to the vincula longa. The dissection, therefore, is quite careful and requires knowledge of the neurovascular anatomy. The cords should only be divided after the neurovascular structures have been identified.

Once the cords have been identified proximally and distally and released from the underlying structures and from the skin, the main cord is divided proximally. This usually corrects the MCP joint contracture and allows full or almost full extension at that joint (**Fig. 8**). The cord is then dissected off the underlying structures using blunt dissection; a periosteal elevator is useful.

After the division of the insertion of the cord into the sides of the A4 pulley, attention is turned to the PIP joint and assessment of how much improvement has occurred just by resecting the cord. It is common to get at least 50% of improvement of the PIP joint contracture at this stage.

Step 3: Persistent Proximal Interphalangeal Joint Contracture

The authors ensure that the skin is not tethered at the sides of the PIP joints by Grayson fascia. After resecting the primary Dupuytren cord and releasing the skin, if correction at the PIP joint is not adequate, the authors perform the following steps[23] in sequence. After each step, a moist swab is applied to the wound, and the PIP joint is gently stretched to break down fine fascial

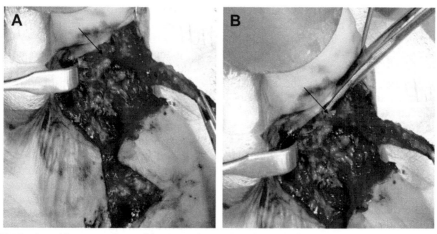

Fig. 7. (*A, B*) Distal cord has extensions of fascia to skin and to the side of the A4 pulley (*arrow*). This is identified and divided.

bands. The stretch is held for a minute or 2 and then correction reassessed. If the correction is full and without any bounce-back, then no further procedure is undertaken, and attention is turned to skin closure. Bounce-back is where the joint resumes its previous bent position when the surgeon releases the digit, rather than remaining in a relaxed, extended position. If there is bounce-back, or the correction is incomplete, then the authors progress to the next step:

1. The authors carefully release taut fascial fibers across the cruciate and A3 pulley; the neurovascular bundle is gently retracted so as not to avulse branches to the vincula.
2. The next step is a transverse split of the tendon sheath just proximal to the A3 pulley. This exposes the flexor tendons. The transverse split

allows fine adhesions over the A3 pulley to be released and is extended to the edges of the sheath. The degree of correction is reassessed.

3. The next step is releasing of the retinacular ligaments. There is usually a stout fascial band, which is identified using a fine-nosed scissors that go underneath these bands, which are then divided. Once again, the degree of correction is reassessed.
4. If there is still incomplete correction, attention is turned to the volar plate. If there is a stout attachment of the proximal end of the volar plate check-rein ligaments, these are identified proximal to the vascular branches that go to the vincula, just at the distal mouth of the A2 pulley, and divided at that location. The volar plate is teased off the proximal phalanx with a Watson Cheyne dissector (narrow elevator). The PIP

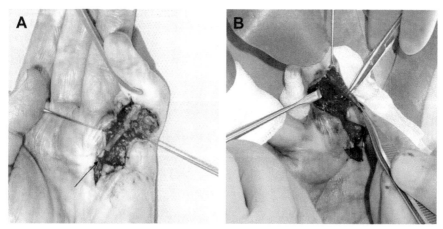

Fig. 8. Photograph (*A*) showing proximal division of the band (*arrow*). The bands is only divided once the neurovascular structures have been identified. (*A*) MCP corrected fully. (*B*) Distal insertion A4.

joint is stretched again, and a decision is made whether or not to go on to the next step. The authors rarely release the accessory collateral ligaments.

5. The final step is arthrolysis of the PIP joint, which may include capsulotomy and/or collateral ligament release. The benefits of proceeding to this additional release are unproved. When operating on a long-standing, severe Dupuytren contracture, abandoning the procedure wherever satisfactory improvement is achieved should be considered, without trying to get the digit fully straight.

Hohendorff and colleagues[24] followed-up 28 patients for just under 2 years and concluded the outcome of severe PIP contracture of over 80° was improved to 29° in most patients after capsuloligamentous release. It has been suggested that the prognosis is poor when surgical release of the PIP joint was required. Beyermann and colleagues[25] found no statistical significance in the outcome between 11 patients with severe contractures undergoing capsuloligamentous release and 32 who did not at 6 months.

Step 4: Assessments After Correction Is Completed

After as much correction as possible is obtained, preliminary hemostasis is obtained while the tourniquet is still inflated. The tourniquet is then released, and a set of observations, each indicating an action, is made as follows:

- Perfusion of the fingertip and skin flaps are assessed to detect areas of reduced blood supply that may lead to necrosis and possible infection (**Fig. 9**). This can be avoided by

ensuring skin flaps have a broad base and wide angles at the apices. If perfusion is not restored, then the skin may be sutured with no tension (to avoid stretching the microcirculation within the flap and thereby occluding the vessels), leaving an open gap (**Fig. 10**), or the compromised skin may be excised and a full-thickness skin graft taken from the antecubital fossa (**Fig. 11**) applied.

- Hemostasis is performed to stop active bleeding and prevent hematoma formation. Care must be taken, however, because the skin in the hand is well vascularized and there will be a gentle ooze that stops with closure of skin and a light pressure dressing. A decision is made on the need for a drain, especially if a patient is on anticoagulation treatment. The authors prefer to use a simple, narrow, soft silastic ribbon as a drain in such a situation.

- The authors record the degree of correction (**Fig. 12**). This is noted as full correction, almost full correction, partial correction but with good improvement, insignificant correction, or no correction, and this is documented in the records. This may modify postoperative care.

- The authors check the degree of extensor lag by performing the tenodesis test (**Fig. 13**). With the wrist in full flexion, any extension lag of the digits, especially at the PIP joint, is noted. The tenodesis test suggests attenuation and stretching of the central slip, which may need to be addressed with changes in the postoperative splinting regimen. Specifically, dynamic splint protection with therapy to help recover of the balance of the extensor mechanism can be used. Even with these precautions, the authors anticipate that there will be a greater loss of correction in those patients

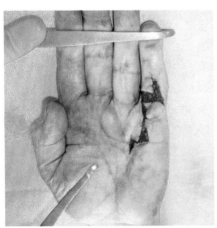 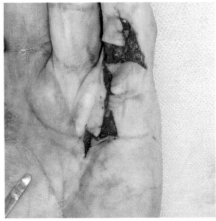

Fig. 9. (*A, B*) Transposed Z-plasty flaps after correction of contracture. The tourniquet is released and the circulation of the finger and flaps assessed.

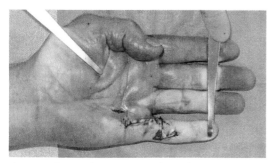

Fig. 10. Closure leaving gaps if needed, rather than suturing the skin under tension.

with an extensor lag present at the end of the operation, and patients are warned of this.

- The authors check the passive flexion range of motion of the distal interphalangeal joint and record this, because a hand therapist can focus on restoring flexion at the distal interphalangeal joint. This occasionally requires release of a tight lateral band.
- The skin gap is assessed, and if this is more than 1.5 cm in the finger, then a full-thickness skin graft (see **Fig. 11; Fig. 14**) is considered to accomplish skin closure without tension. If the gap is less than 1 cm, it can be left open to heal by secondary intention. Gaps larger than 1.5 cm can be tolerated in the palm. If the skin graft is needed, this is taken from the antecubital fossa along the

skin crease, fenestrated, and then sutured in place using an absorbable fine suture (eg, 5-0 Vicryl). The fenestrations allow some drainage to escape and may help avoid formation of a hematoma, which can lift the graft off its bed. Some investigators believe small skin grafts like these function as firebreaks and decrease chance of recurrence.[26,27]

The skin graft should not be quilted, but the gauze dressing should be applied to hold the skin graft against its bed. This involves using fine gauze that loops from back to front over the proximal phalanx and back again, so the gauze forms a loop holding the skin graft in place and in contact with its bed.

Step 5: Closure

Tension in any remaining longitudinal fascia can promote early recurrence. It has been suggested that Z-plasty, or a skin graft, lowers the risk of recurrence by eliminating excess tension in the skin, thereby reducing tension in the fascia attached to that skin.[28]

It is acceptable to leave gaps over the proximal phalanx or in the palm. The authors prefer to leave small gaps in the skin, particularly in the transverse limbs,[29] rather than close skin under tension. The authors reviewed the literature for this article to answer the question regarding whether leaving wounds open led to different outcomes. Seven case series[30–37] reported on 325 patients. A mean extension deficit of 21° was reported in 227 patients managed with an open palm method compared with an extension deficit of 38° in 115 patients managed with full wound closure. This review supports the authors' recommendation at present.

The authors use a nonadherent dressing and loosely fluffed gauze to contour to the skin, and the preference is to use a plaster of Paris extension splint mainly to use as a bandage spreader so the fingers are not squeezed together in the immediate postoperative period, avoiding the development of pressure injuries while the fingers are still anesthetized (**Fig. 15**).

The authors hold the finger straight and use an elasticated plaster strip to lightly push the head of the metacarpals and/or the head of the proximal phalanx against the plaster, thereby maintaining the corrected joint position (**Fig. 16**). Again, this must be applied carefully to avoid undue pressure on soft tissues, which can lead to pressure injury.

POSTOPERATIVE CARE

To ensure sufficient postoperative pain relief, the authors infiltrate local anesthetic in the incisions

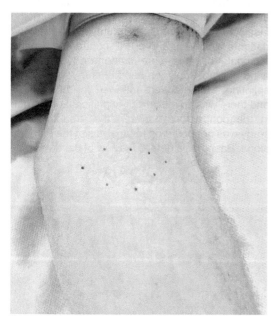

Fig. 11. Skin graft donor site at cubital fossa or the inner side of the arm. The skin edges are approximated with fine absorbable sutures.

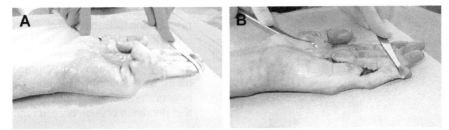

Fig. 12. (*A*) Before and (*B*) after surgical correction. This is documented in the operation record as "Almost full" correction.

at the time of surgery. If the small finger is released, a proximal ulnar nerve block at the wrist also is given.

The aftercare involves checking the circulation, ensuring that it is adequate. Patients have their hands elevated in a sling for approximately an hour to allow the initial hemostasis to occur. An occupational/hand therapy team meets the patient prior to discharge to discuss future management plans, rehearse hand exercises, organize custom-made splints, and provide information leaflets. The exercises allow the tendons to glide and prevent adherence to scar tissue. Exercises commence prior to removal of sutures and include

1. MCP joint range of movement from 0° to 90°
2. Interphalangeal joints full range of movement
3. Abduction and adduction of fingers
4. Opposition of thumb to each finger

The authors encourage enhanced recovery of activities of daily living independence within days of surgery regardless of what is done surgically. This includes early return to most forms of work.

Postoperative care focuses on early recovery of flexion and function, wound healing, and splintage to maintain correction and to stretch surgical scar. The wounds are checked by the clinical staff and monitored; wounds left open are treated just as a split after collagenase injection and the hand is mobilized. Patients are taught how to wash their hand and the open wound and are shown how to use light nonadhesive dressings. Even when a full-thickness skin graft is used, mobilization of the hand is not slowed down. The patient is educated how to hold the proximal phalanx and the overlying skin graft to protect it while recovering PIP joint movement.

At the first occupational therapy appointment, within the first week, the wound is examined, and a custom-made splint (**Fig. 17**) is fabricated. A therapist decides on the design of splint most appropriate for the patient. The splint is usually worn at night so as not to interfere with daily activities. Once the wound has healed, the purpose of the splint is to provide gentle stretch to the surgical scar to help it remodel. The splint may need to be worn for 6 weeks to 3 months. Jerosch-Herold and colleagues[38] performed a multicenter, open, randomized controlled trial to evaluate the effect of night splinting on self-reported function, finger extension, and satisfaction in patients undergoing fasciectomy or dermofasciectomy. A total of 154 patients with MCP and/or PIP contracture from 5 regional hospitals were randomized to receive hand therapy only or hand therapy with night splinting. Patients were followed for 12 months, and there was no statistically significant difference in the contracture between the groups.[38] The study was not powered for analysis of the PIP joint alone. Based on a detailed review of 6 articles[38–44]

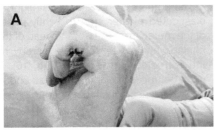
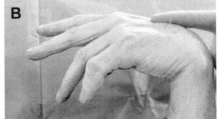

Fig. 13. Tenodesis test for extensor lag at the PIP joint after deformity correction. Holding the wrist in (*A*) full extension and then in (*B*) full flexion, without touching the finger, gives an assessment of extension deficit by looking at the cascade of the fingers and the position of the PIP joint.

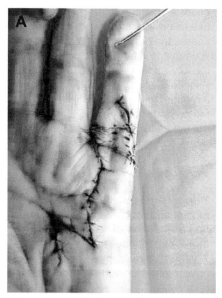
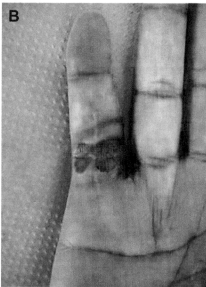

Fig. 14. (*A*) Z-Plasty primarily closed without tension by interposing a firebreak full-thickness skin graft, which is fenestrated to permit escape of hematoma. Skin graft does not alter the mobilization of the hand and finger postoperatively. The patient is shown how to hold the proximal phalanx and the graft while doing exercises for the PIP joint. (*B*) Healed full-thickness skin graft in an Asian patient—note the difference in skin pigmentation.

performed for this article, it seems that splints may not reduce the residual extension deficit in patients with Dupuytren contractures, but further research is likely to have an impact on the conclusions drawn. The authors' current practice is to avoid the use of splints in low-risk patients (straightforward releases of a single joint, for example), but splints are used in patients with more complicated disease, for a variety of reasons.

The sutures are removed at approximately 7 days, the wound is examined for any signs of infection, and advice is given on wound management. Once the sutures are removed, handwashing is permitted as needed even if part of the

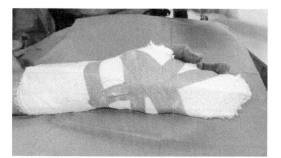

Fig. 16. Bandage and palmar plaster of Paris slab are used to act as a spreader when bandaging fingers after digital fasciectomy. The fingers are held straight and the bandage is used to push the heads of the metacarpals and the head of the proximal phalanx against the plaster, maintaining joint extension. The slab extends from the distal forearm to the tips of the fingers. This prevents maceration and pressure between adjacent fingers and helps maintain correction achieved in the first few days after surgery. Note that the index finger is kept free so the patient is able to function using the thumb and index for the many bimanual tasks of daily living immediately after surgery.

Fig. 15. Pressure sore after bandages removed. This can be avoided by using the plaster slab immediately after surgery to act as a bandage spreader and prevent excessive pressure in the immediate postoperative period when the finger is still numb from the anesthetic.

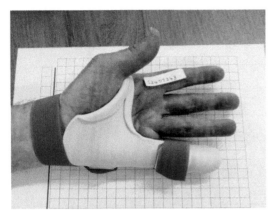

Fig. 17. Custom splint made by the occupational therapist is used at night for the initial few weeks to help stretch surgical scar.

wound is open. Patients are taught how to manage their wounds and provided with nonadherent dressings. Patients are advised to start using their hand as normally as they can.

The therapist advises on massaging the scar using moisturizing cream if the scar and skin require this. This helps reduce dryness, dislodge any scabs, soften the skin, reduce swelling, and warm the tissue. By doing the hand massage, it is easier to carry out the exercises to regain hand function.

An outpatient follow-up appointment at 2 months to 3 months is used to document hand function and note complications and early signs of loss of correction. The authors measure the extension deficit using goniometry and then assess the patients, using photographs if a patient is unable to attend clinic, at a year after surgery to identify recurrent contracture. The authors use a threshold of 20° worsening of contracture from 3 months to 1 year to define recurrence.[45] Further follow-up appointments may be required to assess the need for intervention for other digits or to monitor the status of the operated digit(s).

RECURRENCE

True recurrence after surgery is the reformation of joint contracture after full or almost full correction at the time of surgery (**Fig. 18**).[15] In the authors' experience, this is approximately 12% at 7 years[46] but vastly different recurrences rates have been reported with different definitions of recurrence.

A recent Delphi consensus study, a method of gaining consensus, determined that "more than 20° of contracture recurrence in any treated joint at 1 year post-treatment compared to 6 weeks post-treatment" defines recurrence. In addition, the investigators recommended that "recurrence should be reported individually for every treated joint."[45]

COMPLICATIONS AND MANAGEMENT

Table 2 presents the common complications after limited fasciectomy, based on observational

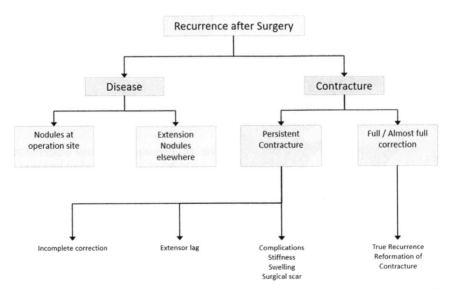

Fig. 18. Flow diagram of the various definitions of recurrence used in the literature. (*Adapted from* Dias JJ, Braybrooke J. Dupuytren's contracture: an audit of the outcomes of surgery. J Hand Surg Br 2006;31(5):520; with permission.)

Table 2
Complications after limited fasciectomy for Dupuytren contracture

Complications	Limited Fasciectomy	Events	Percentage	Minimum	Maximum
Infection[47–60]	6369	183	2.9	0	9.5[59]
Nerve injury[29,47–62]	6558	226	3.4	0	21.4[47]
Vascular complication[29,48–60]	6395	135	2.1	0	10.2[51]
Skin necrosis[47–49,55–59,61]	5296	215	4.1	0	14.7[57]
CRPS[29,47–51,53,55,57–62]	3588	178	5.0	0	19.4[51]
Stiffness[47,51,55]	1465	75	5.1	4.6	10.7[47]
Tendon injury[48,56]	2995	5	0.2	—	—
Amputation[51,55,56,58]	4693	19	0.4	—	—
Other[47,50,52,55,58–60,62]	2654	87	3.3	1.2	50[47]
Total number	6615	—	—	—	—
Number at follow-up	6558	—	—	—	—

studies reporting these complications. The authors did not assume that a complication did not occur if it was not reported in the study when collating published information for this article. Patients need to be advised about these complications and every effort made to avoid, recognize, and mitigate these adverse events. Complications include infection, nerve damage, complex regional pain syndrome (CRPS), and scar-related problems.

In patients with primary disease, the intraoperative complications include digital nerve injury in 3.4% (range, 0.0%–9.5%) and digital artery injury in 2.1% (range, 0%–10.2%). The rate is similar to that previously reported.[63] To avoid dividing the neurovascular structures

1. Beware of the spiral nerve.
2. Avoid cutting cords without identifying the neurovascular structures first.
3. Cut cords a little at a time while rechecking for the neurovascular in between.
4. Ensure dissecting beneath the cords to fully define the neurovascular structures.

Postoperative complications included skin necrosis in 4.1% of cases. This usually does not need intervention or modification of care apart from being alert to infection, which has been reported in 2.9% of cases. Hematoma formation does not cause problems long term and can be reduced by ensuring patients are off anticoagulation medication when possible, leaving parts of the wound open, or using a silastic ribbon drain.

CRPS occurs in 5% of limited fasciectomy cases. The authors treat this seriously with a low threshold to identify it if the hand is swollen and the patient cannot touch the palm with the

fingertips. Management addresses pain, swelling, and movement with frequent monitoring in clinic.

In 1991, McFarlane and colleagues reported amputation rates of 1% of all little fingers that underwent surgery for recurrent disease; this is rare at present.[64–67] The overall rate of serious complications, such as a tendon injury, is 0.2% and loss of the digit is 0.4%.

In 2006, Dias and Braybrooke[15] reviewed the outcomes of surgery in 1177 patients. There was a clear correlation between incidence of each reported complication and the severity of the initial deformity, with a greater deformity having higher complication rates.

SUMMARY

Management of patients with Dupuytren contracture can be challenging, and careful selection of the appropriate procedure, performance of the intervention, and postintervention care are required to usefully improve function. The choice of surgical procedure is based on patients' needs; patients have to bear in mind that surgery is not a cure but an attempt to restore function.

When dealing with a stiff PIP joint, a sequence of releases can be performed to achieve adequate correction. These should be carried in a step-by-step manner with repeated checks and assessment at the end of each step.

The benefits of volar plate release and/or arthrolysis have not been established. The role of minimal goals surgery should be understood and the procedure stopped once adequate correction is achieved without persevering to get full correction.

Small wounds of up to 1.5 cm may be left open in the digits; larger wounds may be left open in the palm to heal by secondary intention.

Early rehabilitation and encouragement of independence with activities of daily living are highly recommended.

REFERENCES

1. Hindocha S, McGrouther DA, Bayat A. Epidemiological evaluation of Dupuytren's disease incidence and prevalence rates in relation to etiology. Hand (N Y) 2009;4:256.
2. Gudmundsson KG, Arngrímsson R, Sigfússon N, et al. Epidemiology of Dupuytren's disease: clinical, serological, and social assessment. The Reykjavik Study. J Clin Epidemiol 2000;53:291–6.
3. Ross DC. Epidemiology of Dupuytren's disease. Hand Clin 1999;15:53.
4. Geoghegan JM, Forbes J, Clark DI, et al. Dupuytren's disease risk factors. J Hand Surg Br 2004;29:423–6.
5. Burge P, Hoy G, Regan P, et al. Smoking, alcohol and the risk of Dupuytren's contracture. J Bone Joint Surg Br 1997;79:206–10.
6. DiBenedetti DB, Nguyen D, Zografos L, et al. Prevalence, incidence, and treatments of Dupuytren's disease in the United States: results from a population-based study. Hand (N Y) 2011;6:149–58.
7. Hueston JT. Table top test. Med J Aust 1976;2:189–90.
8. Heuston JT. The Dupuytren's diathesis. Dupuytren's contracture. London: E & S Livingstone Ltd; 1963. p. 51–63.
9. Hindocha S, Stanley JK, Watson S, et al. Dupuytren's diathesis revisited: evaluation of prognostic indicators for risk of disease recurrence. J Hand Surg Am 2006;31:1626–34.
10. McCann BG, Logan A, Belcher H, et al. The presence of myofibroblasts in the dermis of patients with Dupuytren's contracture a possible source for recurrence. J Hand Surg Br 1993;18:656–61.
11. Tubiana R, Michon J, Thomine JM. Scheme for the assessment of deformities in Dupuytren's disease. Surg Clin North Am 1968;48:979–84.
12. Hindocha S, Stanley JK, Watson JS, et al. Revised Tubiana's staging system for assessment of disease severity in Dupuytren's disease-preliminary clinical findings. Hand 2008;3:80–6.
13. McGrouther DA. The microanatomy of Dupuytren's contracture. Hand 1982;14:215–36.
14. Shewring DJ, Rethnam U. Cleland's ligaments and Dupuytren's disease. J Hand Surg Eur 2014;39:477.
15. Dias JJ, Braybrooke J. Dupuytren's contracture: an audit of the outcomes of surgery. J Hand Surg Br 2006;31:514–21.
16. Moermans JP. Segmental aponeurectomy in Dupuytren's disease. J Hand Surg Br 1991;16:243–54.
17. Shin EK, Jones NF. Minimally invasive technique for release of Dupuytren's contracture: segmental fasciectomy through multiple transverse incisions. Hand 2011;6:256–9.
18. Hueston JT. Limited fasciectomy for Dupuytren's contracture. Plast Reconstr Surg 1961;27:569–85.
19. Logan AM, Brown HG, Lewis-Smith P. Radical digital dermofasciectomy in Dupuytren's disease. J Hand Surg Br Eur 1985;10:353–7.
20. Armstrong JR, Hurren JS, Logan AM. Dermofasciectomy in the management of Dupuytren's disease. J Bone Joint Surg Br 2000;82:90–4.
21. Skoog T. Dupuytren's contracture: pathogenesis and surgical treatment. In: Hueston JT, Tubiana R, editors. Dupuytren's disease. London: Grune & Stratton; 1974. p. 109–17.
22. Short WH, Watson HK. Prediction of the spiral nerve in Dupuytren's contracture. J Hand Surg Am 1982;7:84–6.
23. Curtis RM. Volar capsulectomy of the proximal interphalangeal joint in Dupuytren's contracture. In: Hueston JT, Tubiana R, editors. Dupuytren's disease. London: Grune & Stratton; 1974. p. 135–9.
24. Hohendorff B, Biber F, Sauer H, et al. Die ergänzende Mittelgelenkarthrolyse bei der operativen Behandlung einer Dupuytren'schen Beugekontraktur am Finger. [[Supplementary arthrolysis of the proximal interphalangeal joint of fingers in surgical treatment of Dupuytren's contracture]]. Oper Orthop Traumatol 2016;28:4–11.
25. Beyermann K, Prommersberger KJ, Jacobs C, et al. Severe contracture of the proximal interphalangeal joint in Dupuytren's disease: does capsuloligamentous release improve outcome? J Hand Surg Br 2004;29:240–3.
26. Hueston JT. 'Firebreak' grafts in Dupuytren's contracture. Aust N Z J Surg 1984;54:277–81.
27. Ullah AS, Dias JJ, Bhowal B. Does a 'firebreak' full-thickness skin graft prevent recurrence after surgery for Dupuytren's contracture?: a prospective, randomised trial. J Bone Joint Surg Br 2009;91:374–8.
28. Citron N, Hearnden A. Skin tension in the aetiology of Dupuytren's disease; a prospective trial. J Hand Surg Br 2003;28:528–30.
29. Foucher G, Cornil C, Lenoble E, et al. A modified open palm technique for Dupuytren's disease. Short and long term results in 54 patients. Int Orthop 1995;19:285–8.
30. Cools H, Verstreken J. The open palm technique in the treatment of Dupuytren's disease. Acta Orthop Belg 1994;60:413–20.
31. Zoubos B, Stavropoulos A, Babis C, et al. The McCash technique for Dupuytren's disease: our experience. Hand Surg 2014;19:61.

32. Zachariae L. Operation for Dupuytren's contracture by the method of McCash. Acta Orthop Scand 1970;41:433–8.

33. Shaw DL, Wise DI, Holms W. Dupuytren's disease treated by palmar fasciectomy and an open palm technique. J Hand Surg Br 1996;21:484–5.

34. Schneider LH, Hankin FM, Eisenberg T. Surgery of Dupuytren's disease: a review of the open palm method. J Hand Surg Am 1986;11:23–7.

35. Lubahn JD, Lister GD, Wolfe T. Fasciectomy and Dupuytren's disease: a comparison between the open-palm technique and wound closure. J Hand Surg Am 1984;9A(1):53–8.

36. Guilhen TA, Vieira ABM, de Castro MC, et al. Evaluation of surgical treatment of Dupuytren's disease by modified open palm technique. Rev Bras Ortop 2014;49:31–6.

37. Alonso-Coello P, Oxman AD, Moberg J, et al. GRADE evidence to decision (EtD) frameworks: a systematic and transparent approach to making well informed healthcare choices. 2: clinical practice guidelines. BMJ 2016;353:i2089.

38. Jerosch-Herold C, Shepstone L, Barrett E, et al. Night-time splinting after fasciectomy or dermo-fasciectomy for Dupuytren's contracture: a pragmatic, multi-centre, randomised controlled trial. BMC Musculoskelet Disord 2011;12:136.

39. White JW, Kang SN, Nancoo T, et al. Management of severe Dupuytren's contracture of the proximal interphalangeal joint with use of a central slip facilitation device. J Hand Surg Eur 2012;37:728–32.

40. Larson D, Jerosch-Herold C. Clinical effectiveness of post-operative splinting after surgical release of Dupuytren's contracture: a systematic review. BMC Musculoskelet Disord 2008;9:104.

41. Rives K, Gelberman R, Smith B, et al. Severe contractures of the proximal interphalangeal joint in Dupuytren's disease: results of a prospective trial of operative correction and dynamic extension splinting. J Hand Surg Am 1992;17:1153–9.

42. Ebskov LB, Boeckstyns MEH, Sørensen AI, et al. Results after surgery for severe Dupuytren's contracture: does a dynamic extension splint influence outcome? Scand J Plast Reconstr Surg Hand Surg 2000;34:155–60.

43. Evans RB, Dell PC, Fiolkowski P. A clinical report of the effect of mechanical stress on functional results after fasciectomy for Dupuytren's contracture. J Hand Ther 2002;15:331–9.

44. Glassey N. A study of the effect of night extension SpLintage on post fasciectomy Dupuytren's patients. Br J Hand Ther 2001;6:89–94.

45. Kan HJ, Verrijp FW, Hovius SER, et al. Recurrence of Dupuytren's contracture: a consensus-based definition. PLoS One 2017;12:e0164849.

46. Dias JJ, Singh HP, Ullah A, et al. Patterns of recontracture after surgical correction of Dupuytren disease. J Hand Surg Am 2013;38:1987–93.

47. Weinzweig N, Culver JE, Fleegler EJ. Severe contractures of the proximal interphalangeal joint in Dupuytren's disease: combined fasciectomy with capsuloligamentous release versus fasciectomy alone. Plast Reconstr Surg 1996;97:560–6.

48. van R, Gerbrandy F, Ter L, et al. A comparison of the direct outcomes of percutaneous needle fasciotomy and limited fasciectomy for Dupuytren's disease: a 6-week follow-up study. J Hand Surg Am 2006;31:717–25.

49. Van Giffen N, Degreef I, De Smet L. Dupuytren's disease: outcome of the proximal interphalangeal joint in isolated fifth ray involvement. Acta Orthop Belg 2006;72:671.

50. Stahl S, Calif E. Dupuytren's palmar contracture in women. Isr Med Assoc J 2008;10:445–7.

51. Sennwald GR. Fasciectomy for treatment of Dupuytren's disease and early complications. J Hand Surg Am 1990;15:755–61.

52. Ritchie JFS, Venu KM, Pillai K, et al. Proximal interphalangeal joint release in Dupuytren's disease of the little finger. J Hand Surg Br 2004;29:15–7.

53. Reuben SS, Pristas R, Dixon D, et al. The incidence of complex regional pain syndrome after fasciectomy for dupuytren's contracture: a prospective observational study of four anesthetic techniques: retracted. Anesth Analg 2006;102:499–503.

54. Misra A, Jain A, Ghazanfar R, et al. Predicting the outcome of surgery for the proximal interphalangeal joint in Dupuytren's disease. J Hand Surg Am 2007;32:240–5.

55. McFarlane RM, McGrouther DA. Complications and their management. In: McFarlane RM, McGrouther DA, Flint MH, editors. Dupuytren's disease biology and treatment. Edinburgh (Scotland): Churchill Livingstone; 1990. p. 377–82.

56. Loos B, Puschkin V, Horch RE. 50 years experience with Dupuytren's contracture in the Erlangen University Hospital–A retrospective analysis of 2919 operated hands from 1956 to 2006. BMC Musculoskelet Disord 2007;8:60.

57. Hoet F, Boxho J, Decoster E, et al. Dupuytren's contracture. Review of 326. Operated patients. Ann Chir Main 1988;7:251–5.

58. Coert JH, Nérin JPB, Meek MF. Results of partial fasciectomy for Dupuytren disease in 261 consecutive patients. Ann Plast Surg 2006;57:13–7.

59. Bulstrode N, Jemec B, Smith P. The complications of Dupuytren's contracture surgery. J Hand Surg Am 2005;30:1021–5.

60. Anwar MU, Al Ghazal SK, Boome RS. Results of surgical treatment of dupuytren's disease in women: a review of 109 consecutive patients. J Hand Surg Am 2007;32:1423–8.

61. Vigroux JP, Valentin P. A natural history of Dupuytren's contracture treated by surgical fasciectomy: the influence of diathesis (76 hands reviewed at more than 10 years). Ann Chir Main Memb Super 1992;11:367–74.

62. Citron ND, Nunez V. Recurrence after surgery for Dupuytren's disease: a randomized trial of two skin incisions. J Hand Surg Am 2005;30:563–6.

63. Becker GW, Davis TRC. The outcome of surgical treatments for primary Dupuytren's disease – a systematic review. J Hand Surg Eur 2010;35:623–6.

64. McFarlane RM. Progress in Dupuytren's disease. J Hand Surg Br 1991;16:237–9.

65. Denkler K. Dupuytren's fasciectomies in 60 consecutive digits using lidocaine with epinephrine and no tourniquet. Plast Reconstr Surg 2005;115:802–10.

66. Meathrel KE, Thoma A. Abductor digiti minimi involvement in Dupuytren's contracture of the small finger. J Hand Surg Am 2004;29:510–3.

67. Ebskov LB, Boeckstyns MEH, Sørensen AI, et al. Day care surgery for advanced Dupuytren's contracture. J Hand Surg Br Eur 1997;22:191–2.

Alternative and Adjunctive Treatments for Dupuytren Disease

Paul M.N. Werker, MD, PhD, FEBOPRAS, FEBHS[a],*,
Ilse Degreef, MD, PhD, EBHS[b]

KEYWORDS

- Dupuytren • Radiotherapy • Pharmacotherapy • Firebreak skin graft • Dermofasciectomy

KEY POINTS

- There is a subset of patients that exhibit an aggressive form of Dupuytren disease with unpredictable results and early recurrence after standard treatment.
- Researchers have suggested disease control treatment strategies to slow down the disease process (radiotherapy, tamoxifen, 5-fluorouracil).
- Firebreak skin grafting and dermofasciectomy are used in an effort to reduce the chance of recurrence.
- Lack of the use of clear definitions of recurrence and poor study design (low levels of evidence) hamper the development of unequivocal treatment guidelines.

INTRODUCTION

Dupuytren disease is a common, chronic disease of the elderly in the Western world. Systematic analysis of the available prevalence studies has shown that this varies between 0.6% and 31.0%.[1] Its phenotype is also quite variable and the role of the genotype,[2–4] environmental factors (including lifestyle, leisure habits, and work[5–7]), and associated diseases (diabetes mellitus, epilepsy, and liver disease)[8] is becoming clearer. In a study in which the overall prevalence was more than 20% in people older than 50 years, most people (80%) had only nodules or pits in the palms of their hands without flexion contracture.[9] Only 4% of that population exhibited the picture we as clinicians are so familiar with, showing flexion contractures of 1 or more joints in variable patterns.[10] Only rarely a patient was seen with a Dupuytren diathesis, a term coined by Hueston[11] in the 1960s and that in recent decades has been further elaborated on. In these patients, the disease starts early, is bilateral, has a clear familial trade, often exhibits ectopic disease (Ledderhose disease, Peyronie disease, and/or Garrod pads), develops early recurrence after standard treatment, and more frequently involves the radial side of the hand.[11–13]

Patients with Dupuytren diathesis form the biggest challenge for surgeons, and the standard Dupuytren "tool box" (limited fasciectomy, needle fasciotomy, and collagenase treatment) does not seem to be adequate to provide optimal care with durable results.[14–17] They often need repetitive treatment, and sometimes end up with great functional deficits, disturbed sensibility, or even finger amputations, despite our best efforts.

The purpose of this article was to review what has been attempted or is advocated to try to

Disclosure Statement: The authors have nothing to disclose.
[a] Department of Plastic Surgery, University Medical Center Groningen, University of Groningen, BB81, Hanzeplein 1, Groningen 9713GZ, the Netherlands; [b] Department of Orthopedic Surgery–Hand Unit, University Hospitals Leuven, University of Leuven, Herestraat 49, Leuven B-3000, Belgium
* Corresponding author.
E-mail address: p.m.n.werker@umcg.nl

Hand Clin 34 (2018) 367–375
https://doi.org/10.1016/j.hcl.2018.03.005
0749-0712/18/© 2018 Elsevier Inc. All rights reserved.

control the disease, which is most needed for the aforementioned subgroup of patients. Some of these adjunctive treatments are well known and accepted (although evidence is not strong), whereas others have only been reported once, or have not been investigated thoroughly, and therefore have not become accepted as good alternative approaches. All are presented, using the available evidence to discuss the effectiveness, durability, advantages, and disadvantages of each option. At the end of the article, the authors give a glimpse into the future of the treatment of complex cases.

OVERVIEW OF ATTEMPTS AT EARLY DISEASE CONTROL
Radiotherapy

Ionizing radiation can control cell growth of rapidly proliferating cells by damaging DNA, leading to apoptosis. As such, radiotherapy has been proposed as a therapeutic option for Dupuytren disease. Low-dose radiotherapy (30 Gy) may inhibit fibroblast proliferation and induce an anti-inflammatory effect.[18,19] The radiation is administered in portions of 3 Gy per day on 5 consecutive days, and after a period of approximately 6 weeks the scheme is repeated.

Available evidence on efficacy of radiotherapy in Dupuytren disease is of low quality. The published reports are retrospective studies on patients with mild disease (Tubiana stage N or 1), in which radiotherapy was prescribed with the intent to stabilize or inhibit the progression of Dupuytren disease.[20,21] Zirbs and colleagues[22] reported less progression in a retrospective cohort analysis: 20% instead of an "expected" 50%. Likewise, the earlier report of Betz and colleagues[21] is compared with the same average 50% number, introduced by Millesi[23] in his book in 1981 in a 6-year follow-up group. Only 1 randomized controlled trial (RCT) has examined this issue, reported by Seegenschmiedt and colleagues in 2001.[18] However, they only compared different settings of radiotherapy without an untreated control group. Moreover, only preliminary results after 1-year follow-up were available, and no further data were reported later. All available conclusions on radiotherapy outcomes thus report possible improvement but lack an untreated control group. Therefore, true evidence for the efficiency of radiotherapy in the prevention of Dupuytren contractures is unavailable today, and a long-term possible post-radiotherapy increase in disease progression cannot be excluded.[22] Reported side effects are acute erythema in up to 40% and late skin atrophy in fewer than 10%. Although

no post-radiation malignancies have been reported yet, an absolute 0.02% risk increase is estimated.[24] Salvage surgery is reported to remain safe, although no statistical comparative data or evidence are available. Although the aim of radiotherapy is cell death of myofibroblasts in Dupuytren disease, late radiation fibrosis is a well-known side effect of radiotherapy in general. These long-term effects necessitate a longer follow-up in patients with Dupuytren disease, with respect to effects of radiation on recurrence, progression, and surgical complexity if surgical intervention is ultimately required.

In conclusion, irradiation as a preventive measure for disease progression is inconclusive today. In mild forms, side effects and late malignancy risk must be weighed against the use of radiotherapy. In extreme disease progression, the patient may consider radiotherapy in a multidisciplinary setting with the patient's hand surgeon and radiation oncologist, certainly if surgery may be challenging or is not feasible due to recurrent or extensile Dupuytren contractures. However, because outcome is unsure, even unexpected disease progression after radiotherapy cannot be ruled out as a possible complication as an irradiation side effect.

On balance, radiotherapy should be considered an unproven treatment for early Dupuytren disease due to a scarce evidence base and unknown long-term adverse effects. Well-designed randomized controlled studies are required to confirm the benefits of radiotherapy treatment.

Pharmacotherapy

Pharmaceutical control of myofibroblast activity is an interesting area of translational research that seeks to reduce progression or recurrence of contractures after Dupuytren disease treatment. Conceptually, pharmacotherapy can be applied topically, injected or implanted locally, or administered systemically. Clearly, benefits of possible disease control must outweigh possible risks of treatment, given that Dupuytren disease is a benign entity.[25] Numerous drugs have been suggested, but few level I evidence research studies on pharmacotherapy in Dupuytren disease exist. Treatment options can be categorized as anti-inflammatory drugs (treating Dupuytren disease as an inflammatory process), anti-mitotic drugs (treating Dupuytren disease as a neoplasm), and other pharmacologic targets (eg, hormonal therapy).

Anti-inflammatory drugs
Anti-inflammatory drugs, such as cortisone, interferon, and colchicine, have been suggested for

Dupuytren disease control, but limited evidence is available. Baxter and colleagues[26] first reported on a possible benefit of cortisone in 5 patients in 1946. However, disappointing effects of postoperative *systemic* cortisone was reported 5 years later in 7 of 19 operated patients.[27] Bernstein[28] mentioned a "remission" state in 14 cases after postoperative systemic cortisone treatment without symptoms of recontracture.

Almost 50 years later, Meek and colleagues[29] focused on transforming growth factor (TGF)-beta in fibrosis and advocated further research for clinical immunomodulation in Dupuytren disease. They studied the role of programmed cell death in steroid treatment and found that steroids reduced specific Dupuytren fibroblast proliferation with increasing rates of apoptosis of both fibroblasts and inflammatory cells.[29]

A 97% success rate was reported after *intralesional* steroid injections in 63 patients with mild nodular forms of Dupuytren disease.[30] The nodules softened or flattened temporarily and this was considered disease regression, although recurrence was seen in 50%. Recently, an RCT in needle fasciotomy with steroid injection compared with placebo in 47 patients, demonstrated increased clinical result with improved finger extension and lower retreatment rates in a 6-month follow-up.[31]

Reports on topical cortisone treatment are only expert opinion and case series level of evidence.

On anti-inflammatory drugs other than cortisone, even less evidence is available. In 1992, the administration of colchicine, known to induce collagenase activity and decrease collagen synthesis, was reported in 3 patients with fibrosis. One of them had Dupuytren disease. His tumor size reduced and contracture improved.[32] Oral administration of colchicine improved penile contractures in 24 patients with Peyronie disease. However, the concomitant Dupuytren contractures in these patients, did not improve.[33]

Gamma-interferon is a cytokine produced by T-helper lymphocytes; it is known to decrease fibroblast replication, activation, and collagen production. In a clinical pilot study, gamma-interferon was injected into the nodules of 14 Dupuytren patients and appeared to reduce nodule size and symptoms.[34] However, no further reports on these preliminary observations are available. Interferon-alpha2b appeared to decrease myofibroblast contractility of 3 paired strains of Dupuytren fibroblasts versus control in collagen lattice models.[35]

Anti-mitotic drugs

Anti-mitotic drugs, like 5-FU (5-fluorouracil) and anti-TNF (tumor necrosis factor), have also been suggested for Dupuytren disease control, but again, limited evidence is available. The cytostatic drug 5-FU inhibits thymidylate synthase needed for DNA synthesis. Its inhibitory effect on proliferation and differentiation has been demonstrated in vitro on Dupuytren myofibroblasts.[36] However, an RCT in 15 patients with intraoperative 5-minute topical application of 5-FU failed to show any beneficial effect.[37]

The cytokine TNF, implicated in tumor regression, was shown in vitro as a key regulator of myofibroblast differentiation/activity in early Dupuytren disease, TNF blockade led to downregulation of the myofibroblast. These findings suggest that local injection of anti-TNF may prevent progression of nodules to contractures.[38] However, no clinical trial reports are available.

The literature contains sporadic reports to suggest further research for the use of other antiproliferative drugs to modify the course of Dupuytren disease. A possible short-term beneficial effect of N-sulfonylpyridimide derivative was mentioned, and Amidino-substituted bezimidazo quinolone may exert a nonspecific antiproliferative activity.[39]

Other pharmacologic agents

As androgen receptors are expressed by the myofibroblasts in Dupuytren nodules, the effect of 5 alfa-dihydrotestosterone was investigated on cultured Dupuytren cells in 2003.[40] Fibroblast activation and proliferation increased, with secondary downregulation of the androgen receptors.

Similar in vitro work on Dupuytren myofibroblast contractility on collagen lattices suggested that tamoxifen, a synthetic nonsteroidal antiestrogen known to modulate TGF (beta) production, might be of value in the treatment of Dupuytren disease.[41] This nonsteroidal antiestrogen decreased Dupuytren fibroblast contractility and TGF-beta2 production. In a level I translational clinical trial in high fibrosis diathesis patients with Dupuytren disease, tamoxifen significantly improved short-term outcome of segmental fasciectomy in Dupuytren disease, identified with the Abe score.[42] However, the beneficial effect was lost within 2 years, and the side effects of high-dosage estrogen were not well tolerated in the predominantly male Dupuytren population.

Other pharmaceutical suggestions without clinical trials are numerous.[25] Likewise, numerous topicals are used in Dupuytren treatment, but hardly any trials are reported.

Interposition Materials

To increase the effect of segmental fasciectomy and to isolate the affected skin from the underlying myofibroblasts of Dupuytren tissue, the use of interposing implant materials has been suggested. In 2013, a thin absorbable cellulose implant, shaped to the required firebreak size, was studied in a case control series of 30 patients with a high probability for recurrent disease. The intention was to improve the effect of segmental cord interruption by creating an increased "firebreak" effect with this inert resorbing implant.[43] Finger extension, pain, and patient satisfaction were all significantly better in the cellulose implant group compared with matched controls who did not get the implant. Unfortunately, although it had been successfully used for more than 5 years, cellulose is no longer commercially available as of the publication of this article. Similarly, based on reported lower recurrence rates under a full-thickness skin graft,[44] acellular dermal matrix, which has a common inhibitory effect on underlying myofibroblasts, was studied in 2014.[45] In a retrospective cohort study, 20 patients with open fasciectomy were compared with an experimental group with acellular dermal matrix of 23 in a median follow-up of 1.8 years. Recurrence of contracture was observed in 1 of 23 patients in the group receiving acellular dermal matrix, compared with 5 of 20 in the control group ($P = .045$).

Alternative Surgical Approaches

Variations in incisions
An enormous variety of incisions has been described for limited fasciectomy.[46] However, most surgeons will use either zig-zag (Bruner) incisions and use Y-V plasties to close defects, or longitudinal incisions incorporating Z-plasties at the flexion creases at the time of wound closure. In 1964, McCash[47] described an approach that became quite popular in the United Kingdom. He advocated transverse incisions in the distal palm and along the finger joint creases to access and remove the pathology (**Fig. 1**). The transverse incision in the palm had actually already been used by Dupuytren while performing open fasciotomy in 1833[48] and by Skoog[49] in the 1950s (**Fig. 2**). The incisions give good access to the pathology. An important aspect of the technique is that, after fasciectomy and contracture release, often a skin shortage results, making it impossible to close all wounds. This is not a problem, as McCash[47] has shown: the wounds in the fingers can usually be closed, and the remaining defect in the palm will heal secondarily within 6 to 8 weeks. The technique even carries the advantage that a hematoma will drain easily. Jacobsen and Holst-Nielsen[50] have advocated a combination of the McCash[47] technique and a midlateral ulnar incision for the fasciectomy of the little finger in case of severe

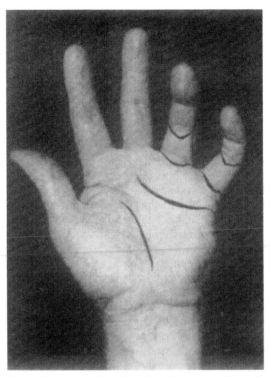

Fig. 1. The planned incision for the open palm technique. Note proximal convexity of incisions at proximal interphalangeal joints. (*From* McCash CR. The open palm technique in Dupuytren's contracture. Br J Plast Surg 1964;17:273; with permission.)

contractures. They describe excellent access to the pathology without any vascular compromise of the flap and wound healing within 3 to 6 weeks (**Fig. 3**). Thirty years later, Tripoli and Merle[51] confirmed the usefulness of the technique, especially in Tubiana stage III and IV cases. They used it in 98 cases and found its application relatively simple, allowing good exposure for correction of severe contractures. They further advocated it as an alternative for dermofasciectomy and even as an option to avoid amputation of badly contracted digits.[51] In contrast to the inventors, these investigators did report vascular compromise of the flap in 1 case, neurovascular injury in 3 cases, and vascular compromise necessitating amputation in 2 cases. Complex regional pain syndrome (CRPS) occurred in 10% of cases and was resolved with conservative measures. No hematomas or infections were encountered.

Skin grafting defects and skin replacements (dermofasciectomy)
As an alternative to leaving the wounds open as in the McCash[47] technique, Ketchum and Hixson[52] has proposed the use of skin grafts to close

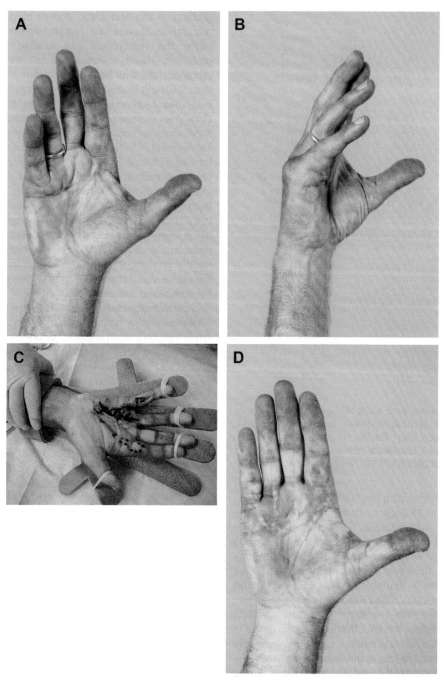

Fig. 2. A 63-year-old man with primary Dupuytren disease of the right index, ring, and little fingers. (*A, B*) Preoperative photographs. (*C*) At the end of the procedure, there was limited fasciectomy using Skoog's approach (transverse incision in the palm and longitudinal with Z-plasty in the little finger and short scar longitudinal for ring finger). The cord in the index finger ray was released by needle fasciotomy. Note the defect in the palm that is left to heal secondarily. (*D*) Photograph of hand 4 weeks postoperatively.

remaining defects. In their view, this not only resulted in faster wound healing, but they also claimed to have seen no recurrences under the grafts following application of this technique in 68 patients between 1970 and 1985. In 8% of cases, they noted extension of the disease outside the full-thickness grafts. In line with Hueston,[44,52] they like to look on the grafts as "firebreaks" to prevent recurrence. Ullah and colleagues[53] tested this concept in a randomized clinical trial in 90 fingers,

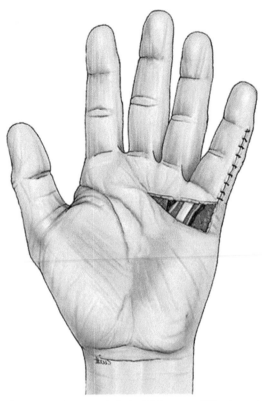

Fig. 3. Jacobsen and Holst-Nielsen modification of the McCash technique. (*From* Tripoli M, Merle M. The "Jacobsen Flap" for the treatment of stages III–IV Dupuytren's disease: a review of 98 cases. J Hand Surg Eur Vol 2008;33(6):780; with permission.)

in which they used a longitudinal incision for fasciectomy. In all fingers, closure with tension-free Z-plasties was possible. However, in approximately half of the cases, they randomly replaced the Z-plasty with a skin graft. The overall recurrence was 12% over 3 years, with no differences between the 2 groups, thereby challenging the findings of Hueston and Ketchum and Hixson.[53]

In the late 1960s, Hueston[11,54–57] drew attention to his view about the effectiveness of skin grafts in the prevention of recurrence and wrote extensively about this and the role of the skin in Dupuytren disease. The "dogma" that resulted from this work was that Dupuytren disease does not recur under a skin graft. This, however, needed to be nuanced after reports started to appear in the 1980s about recurrence under the grafts. In some of these reports, in retrospect, the investigator felt that not all Dupuytren "source" tissue might have been removed.[58] In another case, at reoperation, pathology was found behind the neurovascular bundle.[57] In 1997, Hall and colleagues[59] described the 24 to 100 months of follow-up results of 90 rays in 67 patients who had been treated by dermofasciectomy and skin

grafting. In this and 2 subsequent studies, an 8% recurrence rate was found and in two-thirds of these cases the recurrence was located under the graft.[59,60] These investigators felt that this recurrence rate was nevertheless very much lower than following limited fasciectomy and recommended their technique "for all cases of recurrent Dupuytren's disease requiring reoperation and as a primary procedure when there is significant skin involvement."[59] The dermofasciectomy is performed as follows[58]: all tissues overlying the flexor tendon sheath and the neurovascular bundles are excised including the overlying skin, extending from the distal palmar crease to the distal interphalangeal crease and to the midaxial line on either side of the finger. We usually stop our excision where the pathology ends, which is usually halfway along the middle phalanx, in an effort to preserve some of the native skin if there is no sign of disease (**Fig. 4**). In some cases, this proved too optimistic, and a second dermofasciectomy to the level of the distal interphalangeal joint had to be performed later. The flexor tendon sheath is bared, as are the neurovascular bundles, which are left in their bed unless there is clearly affected tissue deep to them. Leaving the neurovascular bundles in their bed is done to try to preserve as much vascularization to the digit as possible. The authors' personal experience has found that this is only seldom possible. Especially in recurrences, the bundles are usually encased by affected fascia, because Cleland ligaments are often involved.[61,62] Full-thickness skin grafts are preferably taken from the ipsilateral forearm or arm, and donor sites are closed primarily. Grafts from the groin are not used because they typically develop brown pigmentation and hair growth, which is detested by the recipients, and they tend to become bulky. Rents in the flexor sheath, which often occur because the pathology often ends on the A4 pulley, are of no concern: they can be covered by the skin graft, which will bridge them. Logan and colleagues[58] immobilized the skin graft with a tie over bolster and rested the hand in a full hand bandage. We use damp gauzes (wet with normal saline [0.9%]) on top of a paraffin gauze and flush out the space underneath the graft before bandaging the hand. In addition, a plaster splint is applied with the fingers in extension for the first week. This is replaced by a removable thermoplastic splint, which can be removed intermittently for limited flexion and extension exercises.

The convalescence time after dermofasciectomy is longer than after limited fasciectomy, especially in manual workers,[63] as it takes longer for them to return to full flexion and to their work. Delay of return to full flexion is a consequence of the postoperative regimen, because the operated fingers are protected

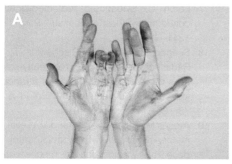
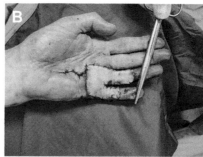
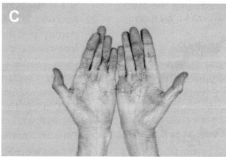

Fig. 4. This 61-year-old man with marked Dupuytren diathesis previously underwent more than 10 procedures (both fasciectomies and collagenase injections). He has significant recurrence in both hands; treatment with dermofasciectomy is planned for the left ring and small fingers as well as the right middle and little fingers. (*A*) Preoperative photograph. (*B*) Immediately following dermofasciectomy and full-thickness skin grafting of the left hand. (*C*) Eight months after surgery of the left hand and 2 months after surgery of the right hand.

in a splint longer than after limited fasciectomy (LF). Once healed, grafts typically become robust and develop sensibility similar to the skin that has been elevated during LF.[58] The most common problem observed following dermofasciectomy and skin grafting was tightness of the radial and ulnar skin graft margin scars, most likely caused by the fact that the graft to normal skin margin runs from proximal-palmar to more dorsal distally. However, none of the patients experienced such discomfort or dissatisfaction that they needed scar revision.[59]

Distant flaps and free flaps in the treatment of Dupuytren disease

In an ultimate attempt to prevent recurrence, Kan and Hovius[64] have applied free flaps after dermofasciectomy in very advanced cases. In 2013, they presented a report on 2 brothers in whom 2 reverse radial forearm flaps were used to cover defects in their hands, and 2 lateral arm flaps were used to reconstruct defects after dermofasciectomy of the soles of their feet. After a follow-up of up to 25 years, no recurrence was noted.[64]

SUMMARY

For the clinical practice of surgeons treating patients with Dupuytren disease, the most relevant findings of this article are as follows:

- There is at present no evidence that radiotherapy is able to prevent progression, while the long-term effects of the treatment are uncertain.
- Pharmacologically, many treatments have been attempted, but no treatment has proved uniformly successful in the short or longer run, and many have had serious side effects. Consequently, no such treatment is at present available for routine use to prevent progression or recurrence.
- Dermofasciectomy and skin grafting may be the best surgical treatment for recurrent cases, especially in patients with a strong diathesis, because a recurrence under a skin graft is only rarely seen. Notwithstanding this, supporting evidence is mostly limited to case series, and the only available RCT did not show a difference between Z-plasties and skin replacement.

REFERENCES

1. Lanting R, Broekstra DC, Werker PM, et al. A systematic review and meta-analysis on the prevalence of Dupuytren disease in the general population of western countries. Plast Reconstr Surg 2014; 133(3):593–603.

2. Dolmans GH, de Bock GH, Werker PM. Dupuytren diathesis and genetic risk. J Hand Surg Am 2012; 37(10):2106–11.

3. Larsen S, Krogsgaard DG, Aagaard Larsen L, et al. Genetic and environmental influences in Dupuytren's disease: a study of 30,330 Danish twin pairs. J Hand Surg Eur Vol 2015;40(2):171–6.

4. Ng M, Thakkar D, Southam L, et al. A genome-wide association study of Dupuytren disease reveals 17 additional variants implicated in fibrosis. Am J Hum Genet 2017;101(3):417–27.

5. Descatha A, Raju K. Dupuytrent's disease and occupation: still a debate? Br J Hosp Med (Lond) 2011; 72(11):655.

6. Descatha A, Bodin J, Ha C, et al. Heavy manual work, exposure to vibration and Dupuytren's disease? Results of a surveillance program for musculoskeletal disorders. Occup Environ Med 2012; 69(4):296–9.

7. Broekstra DC, van den Heuvel ER, Lanting R, et al. Dupuytren disease is highly prevalent in male field hockey players aged over 60 years. Br J Sports Med 2016 [pii:bjsports-2016-096236].

8. Broekstra DC, Molenkamp S, Groen H, et al. A systematic review and meta-analysis on the strength and consistency of the associations between Dupuytren disease and diabetes mellitus, liver disease and epilepsy. Plast Reconstr Surg 2018;141(3):367e–79e.

9. Lanting R, van den Heuvel ER, Westerink B, et al. Prevalence of Dupuytren disease in the Netherlands. Plast Reconstr Surg 2013;132(2):394–403.

10. Lanting R, Nooraee N, Werker PM, et al. Patterns of Dupuytren disease in fingers: studying correlations with a multivariate ordinal logit model. Plast Reconstr Surg 2014;134(3):483–90.

11. Hueston JT. Recurrent Dupuytren's contracture. Plast Reconstr Surg 1963;31:66–9.

12. Abe Y, Rokkaku T, Ofuchi S, et al. An objective method to evaluate the risk of recurrence and extension of Dupuytren's disease. J Hand Surg Br 2004; 29(5):427–30.

13. Hindocha S, Stanley JK, Watson S, et al. Dupuytren's diathesis revisited: evaluation of prognostic indicators for risk of disease recurrence. J Hand Surg Am 2006;31(10):1626–34.

14. Roush TF, Stern PJ. Results following surgery for recurrent Dupuytren's disease. J Hand Surg Am 2000;25(2):291–6.

15. Degreef I, De Smet L. Risk factors in Dupuytren's diathesis: is recurrence after surgery predictable? Acta Orthop Belg 2011;77(1):27–32.

16. van Rijssen AL, ter Linden H, Werker PM. Five-year results of a randomized clinical trial on treatment in Dupuytren's disease: percutaneous needle fasciotomy versus limited fasciectomy. Plast Reconstr Surg 2012;129(2):469–77.

17. Eaton C. Evidence-based medicine: Dupuytren contracture. Plast Reconstr Surg 2014;133(5): 1241–51.

18. Seegenschmiedt MH, Olschewski T, Guntrum F. Radiotherapy optimization in early-stage Dupuytren's contracture: first results of a randomized clinical study. Int J Radiat Oncol Biol Phys 2001;49(3): 785–98.

19. Arenas M, Sabater S, Hernandez V, et al. Anti-inflammatory effects of low-dose radiotherapy. indications, dose, and radiobiological mechanisms involved. Strahlenther Onkol 2012;188(11):975–81.

20. Adamietz B, Keilholz L, Grunert J, et al. Radiotherapy of early stage Dupuytren disease. Long-term results after a median follow-up period of 10 years. Strahlenther Onkol 2001;177(11):604–10.

21. Betz N, Ott OJ, Adamietz B, et al. Radiotherapy in early-stage Dupuytren's contracture. Long-term results after 13 years. Strahlenther Onkol 2010; 186(2):82–90.

22. Zirbs M, Anzeneder T, Bruckbauer H, et al. Radiotherapy with soft X-rays in Dupuytren's disease - successful, well-tolerated and satisfying. J Eur Acad Dermatol Venereol 2015;29(5):904–11.

23. Millesi H. Dupuytren'sche kontraktur. Handchirurgie 1981;1:1500–57.

24. Kadhum M, Smock E, Khan A, et al. Radiotherapy in Dupuytren's disease: a systematic review of the evidence. J Hand Surg Eur Vol 2017;42(7):689–92.

25. Degreef I. Non-operative treatments – pharmacotherapy. In: Warwick D, editor. Dupuytren disease. FESSH instructional course. Troino (Italy): C.G. Edizioni Medico Scientifiche s.r.l; 2015. p. 99–106, 9788871103310.

26. Baxter H, Schiller C, Johnson LH, et al. Cortisone therapy in Dupuytren's contracture. Plast Reconstr Surg (1946) 1952;9(3):261–73.

27. Tilley AR, McDonald G. Cortisone in treatment of Dupuytren's contracture. Treat Serv Bull 1953;8(2):60–2.

28. Bernstein H. The current status of cortisone in postoperative treatment of Dupuytren's contracture. N Y State J Med 1954;54(1):90–2.

29. Meek RM, McLellan S, Reilly J, et al. The effect of steroids on Dupuytren's disease: role of programmed cell death. J Hand Surg Br 2002;27(3): 270–3.

30. Ketchum LD, Donahue TK. The injection of nodules of Dupuytren's disease with triamcinolone acetonide. J Hand Surg Am 2000;25(6):1157–62.

31. McMillan C, Binhammer P. Steroid injection and needle aponeurotomy for Dupuytren contracture: a randomized, controlled study. J Hand Surg Am 2012; 37(7):1307–12.

32. Dominguez-Malagon HR, Alfeiran-Ruiz A, Chavarria-Xicotencatl P, et al. Clinical and cellular effects of colchicine in fibromatosis. Cancer 1992;69(10): 2478–83.

33. Akkus E, Carrier S, Rehman J, et al. Is colchicine effective in Peyronie's disease? A pilot study. Urology 1994;44(2):291–5.

34. Pittet B, Rubbia-Brandt L, Desmouliere A, et al. Effect of gamma-interferon on the clinical and biologic evolution of hypertrophic scars and Dupuytren's disease: an open pilot study. Plast Reconstr Surg 1994; 93(6):1224–35.

35. Sanders JL, Dodd C, Ghahary A, et al. The effect of interferon-alpha2b on an in vitro model Dupuytren's contracture. J Hand Surg Am 1999;24(3):578–85.

36. Jemec B, Grobbelaar AO, Wilson GD, et al. Is Dupuytren's disease caused by an imbalance between proliferation and cell death? J Hand Surg Br 1999; 24(5):511–4.

37. Bulstrode NW, Bisson M, Jemec B, et al. A prospective randomised clinical trial of the intraoperative use of 5-fluorouracil on the outcome of Dupuytren's disease. J Hand Surg Br 2004;29(1):18–21.

38. Verjee LS, Verhoekx JS, Chan JK, et al. Unraveling the signaling pathways promoting fibrosis in Dupuytren's disease reveals TNF as a therapeutic target. Proc Natl Acad Sci U S A 2013;110(10):E928–37.

39. Kraljevic Pavelic S, Sedic M, Hock K, et al. An integrated proteomics approach for studying the molecular pathogenesis of Dupuytren's disease. J Pathol 2009;217(4):524–33.

40. Pagnotta A, Specchia N, Soccetti A, et al. Responsiveness of Dupuytren's disease fibroblasts to 5 alpha-dihydrotestosterone. J Hand Surg Am 2003; 28(6):1029–34.

41. Kuhn MA, Wang X, Payne WG, et al. Tamoxifen decreases fibroblast function and downregulates TGF(beta2) in Dupuytren's affected palmar fascia. J Surg Res 2002;103(2):146–52.

42. Degreef I, Tejpar S, Sciot R, et al. High-dosage tamoxifen as neoadjuvant treatment in minimally invasive surgery for Dupuytren disease in patients with a strong predisposition toward fibrosis: a randomized controlled trial. J Bone Joint Surg Am 2014;96(8):655–62.

43. Degreef I, Tejpar S, De Smet L. Improved postoperative outcome of segmental fasciectomy in Dupuytren disease by insertion of an absorbable cellulose implant. J Plast Surg Hand Surg 2011;45(3):157–64.

44. Hueston JT. Dermofasciectomy for Dupuytren's disease. Bull Hosp Jt Dis Orthop Inst 1984;44(2): 224–32.

45. Terry MJ, Sue GR, Goldberg C, et al. Hueston revisited: use of acellular dermal matrix following fasciectomy for the treatment of Dupuytren's disease. Ann Plast Surg 2014;73(Suppl 2):S178–80.

46. McGrouther DA. Treatment. In: McFarlane RM, McGrouther DA, Flint MH, editors. Dupuytren'd disease, biology and treatment, vol. 5. Edinburgh (Scotland): Churchill Livingstone; 1990. p. 295–310.

47. McCash CR. The open palm technique in Dupuytren's contracture. Br J Plast Surg 1964;17:271–80.

48. Elliot D. The early history of contracture of the palmar fascia. Part 2: the revolution in Paris: Guillaume Dupuytren: Dupuytren's disease. J Hand Surg Br 1988;13(4):371–8.

49. Skoog T. Dupuytren's contracture. Postgrad Med 1957;21(1):91–9.

50. Jacobsen K, Holst-Nielsen F. A modified McCash operation for Dupuytren's contracture. Scand J Plast Reconstr Surg 1977;11(3):231–3.

51. Tripoli M, Merle M. The "Jacobsen flap" for the treatment of stages III-IV Dupuytren's disease: a review of 98 cases. J Hand Surg Eur Vol 2008;33(6): 779–82.

52. Ketchum LD, Hixson FP. Dermofasciectomy and full-thickness grafts in the treatment of Dupuytren's contracture. J Hand Surg Am 1987;12(5 Pt 1):659–64.

53. Ullah AS, Dias JJ, Bhowal B. Does a 'firebreak' full-thickness skin graft prevent recurrence after surgery for Dupuytren's contracture? A prospective, randomised trial. J Bone Joint Surg Br 2009;91(3):374–8.

54. Hueston JT. Digital Wolfe grafts in recurrent Dupuytren's contracture. Plast Reconstr Surg Transplant Bull 1962;29:342–4.

55. Hueston JT. 'Firebreak' grafts in Dupuytren's contracture. Aust N Z J Surg 1984;54(3):277–81.

56. Hueston J. The role of the skin in Dupuytren's disease. Ann R Coll Surg Engl 1985;67(6):372–5.

57. Varian JP, Hueston JT. Occurrence of Dupuytren's disease beneath a full thickness skin graft: a semantic reappraisal. Ann Chir Main Memb Super 1990; 9(5):376–8.

58. Logan AM, Brown HG, Lewis-Smith P. Radical digital dermofasciectomy in Dupuytren's disease. J Hand Surg Br 1985;10(3):353–7.

59. Hall PN, Fitzgerald A, Sterne GD, et al. Skin replacement in Dupuytren's disease. J Hand Surg Br 1997; 22(2):193–7.

60. Armstrong JR, Hurren JS, Logan AM. Dermofasciectomy in the management of Dupuytren's disease. J Bone Joint Surg Br 2000;82(1):90–4.

61. Shewring DJ, Rethnam U. Cleland's ligaments and Dupuytren's disease. J Hand Surg Eur Vol 2013; 39(5):477–81.

62. Zwanenburg RL, Werker PMN, McGrouther DA. The anatomy and function of Cleland's ligaments. J Hand Surg Eur Vol 2014;39(5):482–90.

63. Tonkin MA, Burke FD, Varian JP. Dupuytren's contracture: a comparative study of fasciectomy and dermofasciectomy in one hundred patients. J Hand Surg Br 1984;9(2):156–62.

64. Kan HJ, Hovius SE. Long-term follow-up of flaps for extensive Dupuytren's and Ledderhose disease in one family. J Plast Reconstr Aesthet Surg 2012; 65(12):1741–5.

Comparative Outcomes of Dupuytren Disease Treatment

Paul Binhammer, MD, MSc, FRCSC

KEYWORDS

- Dupuytren • Classification • Assessment • Patient-reported outcome • Fasciectomy • Collagenase
- Needle aponeurotomy

KEY POINTS

- Although staging systems have been historically important, current outcomes focus more on angular correction and patient-reported outcomes.
- Recurrence is defined as a more than 2° increase in the passive extension deficit with a palpable cord compared with that at 3 months after treatment.
- The most frequent comparative outcome studies are between collagenase *Clostridium histolyticum* and needle aponeurotomy. These suggest there is no significant difference in outcomes between these techniques at 1 year to 2 years.

INTRODUCTION

With growing interest in alternatives to surgical excision for Dupuytren disease, and multiple methods available for treatment, a consensus as to definitions and outcomes was essential to compare the available treatment options.

DEFINITIONS

Dupuytren Staging

Dupuytren staging can be conceptualized in 3 terms:

1. Assessment: an aspect that might be measured, for example, degree of contracture or type of disease
2. Scoring system: a system that attempts to quantify the disease by producing a series of numbers or discrete variables
3. Classification: subdivisions into types that are not ordinal[1]

Many methods of assessment have been used in the study of Dupuytren disease, including:

1. Degree of contracture or range of motion (ROM)
2. Disease type based on the localization of pathologic fascia[2]
3. Histology[3]
4. Dupuytren diathesis: bilateral disease, family history of Dupuytren, ectopic lesions, and young age at onset of disease[4]
5. Hand function or disability: Unité Rhumatologique des Affections de la Main (URAM); Disabilities of the Arm, Shoulder and Hand (DASH) questionnaire; and the Michigan Hand Questionnaire (MHQ)[1,5]
6. Rate of recovery/time to return to work[1]
7. Recurrence and progression[6–9]
8. Complications[6]

Scoring systems fall into 5 proposed categories:

1. Severity according to degree of contracture
2. Detailed scoring of every digit
3. Systems that score the severity of the condition or results of surgery into arbitrary categories of excellent/good/fair/poor

Conflict of Interest: There are no conflict of interests.
Financial Disclosures: The author declares no financial interests.
Division of Plastic and Reconstructive Surgery, Sunnybrook Health Sciences Centre, 2075 Bayview Avenue, M1 500, Toronto, Ontario M4N 3M5, Canada
E-mail address: p.binhammer@utoronto.ca

Hand Clin 34 (2018) 377–386
https://doi.org/10.1016/j.hcl.2018.03.006

4. Attempts to predict surgical difficulty
5. Questionnaires based on functional assessment scores[1]

Several investigators have reported arbitrary categorization for their postoperative results, which have failed to become established standards in published literature for Dupuytren disease.[10–15] The British Society for Surgery of the Hand Audit Committee conducted a multicenter study to assess the outcomes of surgery.[16] They used a newly created patient questionnaire with graphics to assess the finger contracture and a classification into mild, moderate and severe to determine a patient's preoperative status. The postoperative status was a patient-reported Likert scale and patient-reported outcome questionnaire.[16]

A well-known scoring system is the Tubiana staging system (TSS). This system uses an algebraic sum of the degree of contracture of the metacarpophalangeal (MP) joint, proximal interphalangeal (PIP) joint, and distal interphalangeal (DIP) joint of a specific affected finger ray. Flexion deformity is measured using a goniometer at the joints. There are 4 stages of increasing severity: 0° to 45°, 45° to 90°, 90° to 135°, and greater than 135° (**Table 1**).[9] Tubiana and colleagues[17] subsequently revised the original staging to include the thumb.[17] Other investigators have proposed additions to TSS to address relevant risk factors with disease severity, including diathesis.[18]

Endpoints or Outcomes

Range of motion
ROM is the most commonly used physical outcome measure in Dupuytren literature. A goniometer is used reliably as a tool to assess active and passive ROM.[19] Inconsistencies in terminology and measurement protocol, however, prevent high-quality evidence for future comparative studies.[19]

ROM for Dupuytren studies can be used in several ways, including:

1. The severity of the initial contracture, reported in degrees
2. The residual contracture postintervention at a particular time period, reported in degrees
3. The amount of contracture correction, determining the difference between preintervention and postintervention at a particular time period. This can be reported in degrees or as a percentage of correction of the deficit.

ROM can be reported for a single joint or for a whole digit incorporating the values of the MCP, PIP, and DIP joints. The extension deficit can be determined actively or passively. The amount of contracture can be reported to give either total passive extension deficit (TPED) or total active extension deficit (TAED) for an individual digit.

Correction of contracture
Correction of contracture can be reported using ROM as indicated by the various measures above. In most studies, however, the results are qualified, with no consistency across the literature, preventing comparisons between studies.[20]

An example of a quantitative definition of correction of contracture is used in the Food and Drug Administration phase 3 studies of *Clostridium histolyticum* (CCH) for the treatment of Dupuytren contracture. In these studies, correction of contracture was defined as "clinically successful" if a reduction in primary joint contracture to 0° to 5° of full extension was achieved 30 days after the last injection[21,22]; however, other investigators have used 15° and some have used 90% to 100% correction.

The value of reporting clear methodology of measurement and results in a comparative fashion is clearly required going forward.[19,20]

Patient-reported outcomes
Patient-reported outcome (PRO) measures involve patients being asked a series of questions, and a score is calculated based on patient response. There are various PROs assessing different outcome measures, which are described.

Disabilities of the arm, shoulder and hand The DASH questionnaire is a validated instrument used to score disabilities of the upper extremities during daily activities.[23–25] The DASH score

Table 1
Original staging of Dupuytren disease by Tubiana

Stage	Deformity
0	No lesion
N	Palmar nodule without presence of contracture
1	TFD between 0° and 45°
2	TFD between 45° and 90°
3	TFD between 90° and 135°
4	TFD >135°

Total Flexion Deformity (TFT) is measured with goniometer at the MP, proximal, and DIP joints.[18]
From Tubiana R. Dupuytren's disease of the radial side of the hand. Hand Clin 1999;15(1):149–59; with permission.

examines a patient's ability to perform multiple dexterous tasks, interference with social and working activities, and sleep disturbance, providing an overall assessment of upper extremity function in the context of disease.[26] The 30-item disability/symptom scale is the main part of the DASH questionnaire concerning patient's health status during the week before. Each item is scaled from 0 to 5; henceforth, the scores are added and transformed into a 100-point scale. The lower the score, the less disability experienced by the patient. The QuickDASH is a shortened 11-item version of the DASH, which is more feasible to complete. It is important to recognize that the DASH does not measure individual hand function. A Rasch modeling analysis (a statistical model transforming PRO to a linear scale) concluded that DASH is still acceptable for use with patients affected by Dupuytren contracture.[27]

Michigan hand questionnaire The MHQ is a 37-item hand-specific outcome questionnaire consisting of 6 domains: overall hand function, activities of daily life, pain, work performance, aesthetics, and patient satisfaction. The MHQ has been validated for a variety of hand conditions, inclusive of Dupuytren disease.[5] Patients are asked to answer each question from 1 to 5. Each domain is based on a score of 0 to 100, with 0 the worst score and 100 the best.[5]

Unité rhumatologique des affections de la main URAM is an outcome assessment tool specifically for patients with Dupuytren disease. The URAM scale is a 9-item patient-reported questionnaire with total scores for Dupuytren disease–associated disability ranging from 0 (best) to 45 (worst). Higher scores indicate poorer functional outcome.[28] The URAM scale has been evaluated for reliability and responsiveness with several studies.[29–31]

Pain visual analog scale Patients are asked to rate the severity of the pain they experienced during a particular event, for example, an injection, on a visual analog scale (VAS). This is a line on a paper with the scale rated from 0 (indicative of no pain) to 10 (indicative of worst pain). Patients mark on the line their response and an exact measure of distance is made and recorded.[32] VAS can be used to assess other issues where the endpoints of the line are defined for that issue.

Recurrence
Recurrence has been used in many different ways, including, but not limited to, failure of surgical joint contracture release, disease recurrence within the

surgical area (with or without joint contracture), and disease anywhere within the same ray postsurgery.[16]

A recent study looking at rates of contracture correction and recurrence reviewed 218 studies, of which 21 met their study inclusion criteria. Most studies reviewed reported results in a qualitative fashion preventing comparison. The investigators concluded that clear definitions of correction of contracture and recurrence are required.[20]

To this end, an international conference was held in 2013 after initial online questionnaires using Delphi methodology. The consensus was that:

1. The presence of disease alone without contracture did not constitute recurrence.
2. Recurrence was associated with an individual joint and not a total ray.
3. Time 0 is between 6 weeks and 3 months.
4. Recurrence is a PED of more than 20° for at least 1 treated joint, in the presence of a palpable cord, compared with the result obtained at time 0.[33]

At this same conference, it was determined that the TSS was considered inappropriate for reporting recurrence. The long-term value of staging Dupuytren disease in clinical studies seems to be diminishing, although not gone.[34]

PUBLISHED COMPARATIVE OUTCOMES STUDIES
Surgery Versus Needle Aponeurotomy

Two studies, a randomized controlled study (RCT) and an observational study, have compared the effectiveness of limited fasciectomy (LF) and percutaneous (NA) for Dupuytren contracture.[25,35]

In the RCT study, there were 166 rays: 88 rays in the NA group and 78 rays in the LF group. The inclusion criteria were a PED of at least 30° in a finger and a clearly defined pathologic cord in the palmar fascia.[25] Patients who were enrolled were followed-up 1 week and 6 weeks post-treatment. From weeks 1 to 5, patients were asked to fill out the DASH questionnaire, followed by a satisfaction questionnaire and complication checks at week 6. Study outcomes show that patients treated with NA reported less discomfort after treatment. DASH scores were also significantly lower in the NA group in the first 5 weeks post-treatment.

In a follow-up publication to this RCT, the investigators presented the 5-year recurrence rates, defined as an increase in extension deficit greater or equal to 30° compared with the results at 6 weeks.[36] The recurrence rate in the NA group was significantly greater than in the LF group, and recurrence occurred significantly sooner in the NA group. Recurrence was not associated with any features of Dupuytren diathesis. Older age at the time of treatment significantly decreased the recurrence rate. Patients receiving LF were significantly more satisfied at 5 years with their treatment than those with NA, and this was significantly associated with recurrence. There were 45 recurrences in the NA group. Twelve chose no treatment, 7 chose LF, and 26 chose to repeat NA. In the LF group, there were 9 recurrences: 4 chose to have NA and 5 declined further treatment. None of the LF patients chose to have retreatment with LF.

In the weighted observational study, among the total eligible patients (n = 293), 78 were in the NA group whereas 215 were in the LF group.[35] On average, patients had a follow-up duration of 10 weeks (range 6–12 weeks). The impact of NA and LF on patient-reported hand function was assessed using the MHQ. This study found that among mild to moderate affected digits, NA reduced contractures as effectively as LF in clinical practice. NA had greater MHQ subscores and shorter recovery times and showed significantly lower rate of mild complications.

Surgery Versus Collagenase

There is 1 study that compared clinical results of collagenase CCH and LF. This observational multicenter study used a propensity score to minimize confounding by indication bias[34]; 104 patients were treated with CCH, and 114 were treated with LF. Primary outcome was the degree of TAED at follow-up visits between 6 weeks and 12 weeks postintervention. Secondary outcomes included whether affected joints achieved clinical improvement (defined as >50% reduction from baseline contracture), adverse events, and MHQ. The degree of residual contracture in the 2 treatment arms was not significantly different at the MP joint level, whereas the affected PIP joints were worse in the CCH group compared with the LF group. Patients in the CCH group reported larger and quicker functional improvements as demonstrated by greater MHQ scores. The patients in the CCH group were more satisfied with their finger mobility and hand function than patients in the LF group. The CCH group had significantly better work performance and greater satisfaction at follow-up than the LF group.

Collagenase Clostridium histolyticum versus needle aponeurotomy

There are 3 studies comparing CCH and NA.[37–39] The first was a single-blinded RCT comparing the efficacy of CCH and NA for contracture of the MP joint.[37] The inclusion criteria was a contracture of 20° or more. A cycle of treatment included 1 visit in the NA group, 2 visits in the CCH group, a 7-day follow-up, and a blinded follow-up after 1 year. The primary outcome was a straight finger, defined as reduction in extension deficit in the affected MP joint to 5°. Secondary outcomes were PROs and the presence of complications. CCH patients were found to have significantly greater procedural pain than NA. Final 1-year follow-up results showed significant improvement from baseline in both treatment arms; however, no significant differences were found between treatment after 1 year in terms of reduction in MP contracture or URAM score.

In a second RCT comparing CCH and NA, patients were included with primary Dupuytren contracture, excluding the thumb, with a palpable cord and a total extension deficit from 30° to 135° with less than 60° in the PIP joint.[38] There were 45 patients treated with NA and 38 with collagenase injections. Patients were seen before treatment, and 3 months and 1 year post-treatment. The primary outcome was the degree of total extension deficit. Secondary outcomes were QuickDASH, URAM, recurrence (defined as ≥20° of extension loss between the 3-month and 12-month time points), complications, and pain VAS scores. Reduction of contracture by NA and CCH were similar at 3-month and 12-month follow-ups. Analysis showed that QuickDASH and URAM scores did not differ significantly between the groups before the treatment or at 3 months or 12 months. VAS treatment pain scores at the time of treatment were greater for the CCH group than the NA group at 3 months but not subsequently. Correction of MP joints was maintained at 1 year; however, PIP joint contracture corrections were not maintained in either group.

A third RCT study compared CCH and NA treatment of PIP contractures with a 2-year follow-up. Inclusion criteria were a 20° or more PIP joint PED and a well-defined cord[39]; 50 patients were recruited. There were 29 patients in the CCH group and 21 patients in the NA group. Patients were seen at day 30, at 1 year, and at 2 years. The primary outcome was clinical improvement defined as a reduction in contracture of greater than or equal to 50% from baseline. Secondary outcomes included changes in PIP joint contracture, pulp-to-palm distance, tabletop test, DASH score, clinical success defined as 5° or less PIP joint PED, recurrence defined as 20° or greater PIP joint PED, adverse events, and complications. After 30 days, all NA patients and 89% of CCH patients had clinical improvement. At 2 years, 6 of 19 NA patients and 2 of 24 CCH patients maintained clinical improvement without statistical difference. Transient complications were significantly higher after CCH than NA. Other secondary outcomes remained the same with both groups.

Limited fasciectomy versus dermofasciectomy

In this RCT study of 79 patients, LF with Z-plasty closure was compared with dermofasciectomy with full-thickness skin grafting.[40] Patients with a 30° or greater contracture of the PIP joint were randomized, after full correction and confirmation that the skin over the proximal phalanx could be easily closed, to have either a firebreak skin graft or Z-plasty closure. The primary outcomes of this study were recurrence, ROM, and complications. Patients were assessed at 3 months, 6 months, 12 months, 24 months, and 36 months. There was no clear definition of recurrence in this study, but it was reported that over 3 years there was recurrence at the PIP joint in 5 Z-plasty and 6 skin graft patients, without significant statistical difference. All MCP contractures were corrected fully, whereas PIP deformities were corrected to a mean of 6° with no difference between groups. Groups were comparable in terms of grip strength, ROM, and disability at follow-up.

Modified Bruner Versus Z-plasty

This pseudo-RCT study looked at whether the design of the skin incision affects recurrence rates comparing longitudinal incision with Z-plasty closure with a modified Bruner incision closed by Y-V plasties.[41] Recurrences were defined as any new nodule in the operative field under the flaps. Patients were eligible for entry if they had Dupuytren disease in 1 ray only and any degree of resultant contracture. At 2-year follow-up there were 46 modified Bruner incision and 33 Z-plasties available for evaluation. Secondary outcomes included extension, any complications, algodystrophy, and digital nerve injury. Recurrence rates were not significantly different, 15 in the modified Bruner group compared with 6 in the Z-plasty group. There were no significant differences in any of the secondary outcomes.

Direct Closure Versus Z-plasty

A prospective trial was conducted to test the hypothesis that recurrence rates were reduced if tension is reduced in the skin after fasciotomy.[42] The inclusion criteria were a single cord contracture of a single ray confined to the palm and affecting only the MCP joint; 27 patients were enrolled and were assigned in strict alternation. Patients either had excision through a transverse palmar incision with direct closure, or a longitudinal incision with closure using a Z-plasty. The primary outcome was recurrence defined as the reappearance of Dupuytren tissue in the operative field. At 2 years, 7 of 14 direct closure and 2 of 13 Z-plasty patients had recurrence. The investigators reported statistical significance at follow-up, but it should be noted they set a significance level at $P<.1$, rather than the traditional $P<.05$.

Open Palm Technique Versus Full-Thickness Skin Graft

A prospective study of 30 patients undergoing LF split the patients into 2 groups.[43] The first 10 patients had an open palm technique in which diseased tissue was excised through a transverse palmar incision left to heal secondarily. The second 20 patients had the open palm covered with a full-thickness hypothenar skin graft. Primary outcome was not defined. Patients were compared for ROM, function, appearance, patient satisfaction, joint contractures, recurrence, time to healing, quality of soft tissue, and DASH. The average follow-up was 3.5 years for the open palm group and 2.7 years for the skin graft group. Time to healing and soft tissue outcome were significantly better for the skin graft group. Recurrence was not defined in the study, and it is not clear if there was a significant difference between the groups.

Needle aponeurotomy plus steroid versus needle aponeurotomy alone

A 2014 RCT study, 44 participants were randomized to either NA group (n = 21) or NA combined with triamcinolone acetonide injection (NATI) (n = 23).[44] Inclusion criteria consisted of at least 1 joint contracture of 20° or more. Primary outcome measure was TAED, which was compared on various time scales (months) after treatment. Analysis of the results showed NATI was associated with lower TAED for up to 2 years.

Limited fasciectomy versus percutaneous aponeurotomy and lipofilling

This RCT study compared LF to percutaneous aponeurotomy and lipofilling (PALF) in 80 patients.[45] Dupuytren contracture patients were included if they met the inclusion criteria of having a flexion contracture of at least 20° at the MP joint, at least 30° at the PIP joint, or both. Patients were measured at baseline and at 2 weeks, 3 weeks, 6 months, and 1 year postoperatively. The primary outcomes were contracture correction and convalescence time. Analysis of their results showed no significant differences in contracture correction, with both groups having full MP joint extension at

Table 2
Study comparatives, endpoints or outcomes, study type, study duration, total sample size, and key points of results

Comparative Study	Endpoints or Outcomes Used	Study Type	Study Duration	Total (N)	Results Key Points
Surgery vs NA[25]	1. Total PED 2. Patient satisfaction 3. DASH 4. Complication rate	RCT	6-wk	166 rays: 88 NA,78 LF	NA has less pain and better DASH scores.
Surgery vs NA[36]	1. Recurrence (increase of TPED >30°) 2. Patient satisfaction 3. Flexion 4. Sensibility	RCT	5 y	93 patients: LF: 41, NA: 52	1. Recurrence rates after 5 y higher in the NA group than LF. 2. Older age at treatment decreases recurrence rate.
Surgery vs NA[35]	1. Total residual extension deficit 2. MHQ 3. Complications	Observational study	6–12 wk post-treatment	293 patients: 78 NA, 215	1. No difference in correction mild to moderate 2. NA report better MHQ
Surgery vs CCH[34]	1. Degree of residual contracture 2. Clinical improvement with affected joints (>50% reduction from baseline contracture) 3. Adverse events 4. PROs a. MHQ	Comparative study	6–12 wk post-treatment	218 subjects: 104 CCH, 114 LF	1. PIP joints clinical improvement worse for CCH 2. No difference in clinical improvement for MP 3. CCH group better MHQ values

CCH vs NA[37]	1. Reduction in extension deficit in the affected MCP joint to 5°
	2. PROs
	  a. VAS pain scale
	  b. URAM
	3. Complications
		RCT	1 y	140 patients: 69 CCH, 71 NA	1. No difference CCH vs NA in correction of contractures
					2. No difference in URAM
					3. CCH VAS pain was greater

CCH vs NA[38]	1. Degree of total extension deficit
	2. PROs
	  a. URAM
	  b. VAS pain scale
	  c. QuickDASH
	3. Recurrence
	4. Complications
		RCT	1 y	83 patients: 45 NA, 38 CCH	1. No difference in reduction of contracture
					2. No difference in QuickDASH and URAM
					3. Treatment pain was greater in CCH
					4. PIP joint corrections not maintained in either group

Study	Outcomes	Design	Follow-up	Patients	Findings
CCH vs NA[39]	1. Clinical improvement (reduction in contracture ≥50% from baseline) 2. PIP joint contracture 3. Pulp-to-palm distance 4. Tabletop test 5. Clinical success (≤5° PIP joint PED) 6. Recurrence (≥20° PIP joint PED) 7. Adverse events 8. Complications 9. DASH	RCT	2 y	50 patients	1. No difference in clinical improvement contracture 2. CCH led to higher transient complications
Modified Bruner vs Z-plasty[41]	1. Recurrence 2. Extension 3. Complications 4. Algodystrophy 5. Digital Nerve Injury	RCT	2 y	46 patients in modified Bruner 33 patients in Z-plasty	No difference in recurrence rate
Direct closure vs Z-plasty[42]	1. Recurrence 2. Complications	Prospective trial	1–2 y	27 patients: 14 direct closure, 13 Z-plasty	No difference at $P<.05$
Open palm technique vs skin graft[43]	1. ROM 2. Function 3. Appearance 4. Patient satisfaction 5. Joint contractures 6. Recurrence 7. Time to healing 8. Quality of soft tissue skin 9. DASH	Prospective trial	Average follow-up: Synthesis: 2.7 y; Open palm: 3.5 y	30 patients: 10 in open palm technique, 20 in synthesis of surgical technique	1. Open palm technique takes longer to heal. 2. Skin graft leads to better soft tissue quality. 3. Not clear if there was a difference in recurrence
LF vs DF[40]	1. Recurrence 2. Correction of contractures 3. Complications 4. ROM	RCT	3 y	79 patients: 39 DF, 40 LF	1. No significant difference in recurrence rates 2. No difference in correction of contractures
NA steroid vs NA (no steroid)[44]	1. TAED 2. Length of time from initial procedure to retreatment	RCT	6–53 mo from initial procedure	44 participants: 21 NA, 23 NATI	Triamcinolone injections combined with NA associated with lower TAED for up to 2 y

LF vs PALF[45]	1. Correction of contractures
	2. Convalescence time
	3. PROs
	  a. QuickDASH
	4. Recurrence rates
	  a. Complication
		RCT	1 y	80 patients: 40 LF, 40 PALF	No significant differences in contracture correction

1-year follow-up. PALF-treated hands experienced quicker healing and quicker return to their daily activities and were able to make a full fist earlier than the LF-treated hand group. Recurrence was also not significant at 1 year between groups. QuickDASH improved significantly in both groups.

SUMMARY

Staging systems for Dupuytren disease have played an important role in studies in the past. Although many investigators have created their own staging systems, few have survived the test of time. TSS has been retained in the literature and some investigators have sought to modify it.

Contemporary studies have largely moved away from staging systems, looking at changes in extension deficit and PROs. There is a need for investigators, however, to be clear about how the extension deficit has been calculated. Recent efforts at reaching consensus about the term recurrence have been successful in defining this as 20° greater than the deficit at time 0 with evidence of a Dupuytren cord.

Outcome studies for isolated MCP joint contractures indicate there is no significant improved outcome with CCH compared with NA. At the PIP joint, there is a suggestion that NA is better than CCH; however, this was only evaluated in 1 study.

Comparing NA and LF, 2 studies have shown that NA has a quicker recovery. The 1 long-term RCT comparing LF and NA demonstrates a higher recurrence rate for NA, but this effect decreases for older patients. It is suggested that NA is more preferred intervention in older patients.

A comprehensive, evidence-based treatment algorithm for the management of Dupuytren disease is yet to be determined, but from the few comparative outcomes studies available (**Table 2**), it might be suggested that:

1. Surgery should be used in younger patients to decrease recurrence rates.
2. Surgery has lower recurrence rates.
3. Recurrence rates are lower for older patients.
4. NA recurrence rates are lower in older patients.
5. Patients experience less pain and quicker recovery with NA compared with CCH compared with surgery.
6. Advantages of CCH over NA have not been definitively demonstrated.

ACKNOWLEDGMENTS

The author wishes to thank Michael Hong, BSc, for his assistance with this article.

REFERENCES

1. Akhavani MA, McMurtrie A, Webb M, et al. A review of the classification of Dupuytren's disease. J Hand Surg Eur Vol 2015;40(2):155–65.
2. Sennwald GR. Fasciectomy for treatment of Dupuytren's disease and early complications. J Hand Surg 1990;15(5):755–61.
3. Luck JV. Dupuytren's contracture; a new concept of the pathogenesis correlated with surgical management. J Bone Joint Surg Am 1959;41-A(4):635–64.
4. Hueston JT. Recurrent Dupuytren's contracture. Plast Reconstr Surg 1963;31:66–9.
5. Chung KC, Hamill JB, Walters MR, et al. The Michigan Hand Outcomes Questionnaire (MHQ): assessment of responsiveness to clinical change. Ann Plast Surg 1999;42(6):619–22.
6. Becker GW, Davis TRC. The outcome of surgical treatments for primary Dupuytren's disease–a systematic review. J Hand Surg Eur Vol 2010;35(8):623–6.
7. Shaw DL, Wise DI, Holms W. Dupuytren's disease treated by palmar fasciectomy and an open palm technique. J Hand Surg Br 1996;21(4):484–5.
8. Westacott DJ, Smith EW, Nwachukwu IA. A novel method for community monitoring of flexion contracture in Dupuytren's disease. Ann R Coll Surg Engl 2014;96(3):240.
9. Tubiana R, Michon J, Thomine JM. Scheme for the assessment of deformities in Dupuytren's disease. Surg Clin North Am 1968;48(5):979–84.
10. Woodruff MJ, Waldram MA. A clinical grading system for Dupuytren's contracture. J Hand Surg Edinb Scotl 1998;23(3):303–5.
11. Einarsson F. On the treatment of Dupuytren's contracture. Acta Chir Scand 1946;93(1):1–22.
12. Mcindoe A, Beare RL. The surgical management of Dupuytren's contracture. Am J Surg 1958;95(2):197–203.
13. Davis JE. On surgery of Dupuytren's contracture. Plast Reconstr Surg 1965;36(3):277–314.
14. Honner R, Lamb DW, James JI. Dupuytren's contracture. Long term results after fasciectomy. J Bone Joint Surg Br 1971;53(2):240–6.
15. Figus A, Britto JA, Ragoowansi RH, et al. A clinical analysis of Dupuytren's disease of the thumb. J Hand Surg Eur Vol 2008;33(3):272–9.
16. Dias JJ, Braybrooke J. Dupuytren's contracture: an audit of the outcomes of surgery. J Hand Surg Edinb Scotl 2006;31(5):514–21.
17. Tubiana R, Leclercq C, Hurst L, et al. Dupuytren's disease. 1st Edition. CRC Press; 2000.
18. Hindocha S, Stanley JK, Watson JS, et al. Revised Tubiana's staging system for assessment of disease severity in Dupuytren's disease-preliminary clinical findings. Hand (N Y) 2008;3(2):80–6.

19. Pratt AL, Ball C. What are we measuring? A critique of range of motion methods currently in use for Dupuytren's disease and recommendations for practice. BMC Musculoskelet Disord 2016;17:20.

20. Werker PMN, Pess GM, van Rijssen AL, et al. Correction of contracture and recurrence rates of Dupuytren contracture following invasive treatment: the importance of clear definitions. J Hand Surg 2012;37(10):2095–105.e7.

21. Hurst LC, Badalamente MA, Hentz VR, et al. Injectable collagenase clostridium histolyticum for dupuytren's contracture. N Engl J Med 2009;361(10): 968–79.

22. Gilpin D, Coleman S, Hall S, et al. Injectable collagenase Clostridium histolyticum: a new nonsurgical treatment for Dupuytren's disease. J Hand Surg 2010;35(12):2027–38.e1.

23. Hudak PL, Amadio PC, Bombardier C. Development of an upper extremity outcome measure: the DASH (disabilities of the arm, shoulder and hand) [corrected]. The Upper Extremity Collaborative Group (UECG). Am J Ind Med 1996;29(6): 602–8.

24. Beaton DE, Wright JG, Katz JN, Upper Extremity Collaborative Group. Development of the Quick-DASH: comparison of three item-reduction approaches. J Bone Joint Surg Am 2005;87(5): 1038–46.

25. van Rijssen AL, Gerbrandy FSJ, Ter Linden H, et al. A comparison of the direct outcomes of percutaneous needle fasciotomy and limited fasciectomy for Dupuytren's disease: a 6-week follow-up study. J Hand Surg 2006; 31(5):717–25.

26. Budd HR, Larson D, Chojnowski A, et al. The Quick-DASH score: a patient-reported outcome measure for Dupuytren's surgery. J Hand Ther 2011;24(1): 15–20 [quiz: 21].

27. Forget NJ, Jerosch-Herold C, Shepstone L, et al. Psychometric evaluation of the Disabilities of the Arm, Shoulder and Hand (DASH) with Dupuytren's contracture: validity evidence using Rasch modeling. BMC Musculoskelet Disord 2014;15:361.

28. Beaudreuil J, Allard A, Zerkak D, et al. Unité Rhumatologique des Affections de la Main (URAM) scale: development and validation of a tool to assess Dupuytren's disease-specific disability. Arthritis Care Res 2011;63(10):1448–55.

29. Bernabe B, Lasbleiz S, Gerber R, et al. URAM scale for disability assessment in Dupuytren's disease: A comparative study of its properties. Annals of Physical and Rehabilitation Medicine 2012; 55(n° S1):e65.

30. Bernabe B, Lasbleiz S, Gerber R, et al. URAM scale for functional assessment in Dupuytren's disease: a comparative study of its properties. Joint Bone Spine 2014;81(5):441–4.

31. Rodrigues JN, Zhang W, Scammell BE, et al. What patients want from the treatment of Dupuytren's disease–is the Unité Rhumatologique des Affections de la Main (URAM) scale relevant? J Hand Surg Eur Vol 2015;40(2):150–4.

32. Badalamente M, Coffelt L, Elfar J, et al. Measurement scales in clinical research of the upper extremity, part 2: outcome measures in studies of the hand/wrist and shoulder/elbow. J Hand Surg 2013;38(2): 407–12.

33. Felici N, Marcoccio I, Giunta R, et al. Dupuytren contracture recurrence project: reaching consensus on a definition of recurrence. Handchir Mikrochir Plast Chir 2014;46(6):350–4.

34. Zhou C, Hovius SER, Slijper HP, et al. Comparative effectiveness of collagenase injection for dupuytren contracture. In: dupuytren disease and related diseases - the cutting edge. Cham (Switzerland): Springer; 2017. p. 259–70.

35. Zhou C, Selles RW, Slijper HP, et al. Comparative effectiveness of percutaneous needle aponeurotomy and limited fasciectomy for dupuytren's contracture: a multicenter observational study. Plast Reconstr Surg 2016;138(4): 837–46.

36. van Rijssen AL, ter Linden H, Werker PMN. Five-year results of a randomized clinical trial on treatment in Dupuytren's disease: percutaneous needle fasciotomy versus limited fasciectomy. Plast Reconstr Surg 2012;129(2):469–77.

37. Strömberg J, Ibsen-Sörensen A, Fridén J. Comparison of treatment outcome after collagenase and needle fasciotomy for dupuytren contracture: a randomized, single-blinded, clinical trial with a 1-year follow-up. J Hand Surg 2016;41(9): 873–80.

38. Scherman P, Jenmalm P, Dahlin LB. One-year results of needle fasciotomy and collagenase injection in treatment of Dupuytren's contracture: a two-centre prospective randomized clinical trial. J Hand Surg Eur Vol 2016;41(6):577–82.

39. Skov ST, Bisgaard T, Søndergaard P, et al. Injectable collagenase versus percutaneous needle fasciotomy for dupuytren contracture in proximal interphalangeal joints: a randomized controlled trial. J Hand Surg 2017;42(5):321–8.e3.

40. Ullah AS, Dias JJ, Bhowal B. Does a "firebreak" full-thickness skin graft prevent recurrence after surgery for Dupuytren's contracture?: a prospective, randomised trial. J Bone Joint Surg Br 2009; 91(3):374–8.

41. Citron ND, Nunez V. Recurrence after surgery for Dupuytren's disease: a randomized trial of two skin incisions. J Hand Surg Edinb Scotl 2005;30(6): 563–6.

42. Citron N, Hearnden A. Skin tension in the aetiology of Dupuytren's disease; a prospective trial. J Hand Surg Edinb Scotl 2003;28(6):528–30.

43. Skoff HD. The surgical treatment of Dupuytren's contracture: a synthesis of techniques. Plast Reconstr Surg 2004;113(2):540–4.

44. McMillan C, Binhammer P. Steroid injection and needle aponeurotomy for Dupuytren disease: long-term follow-up of a randomized controlled trial. J Hand Surg 2014;39(10):1942–7.

45. Kan HJ, Selles RW, van Nieuwenhoven CA, et al. Percutaneous Aponeurotomy and Lipofilling (PALF) versus limited fasciectomy in patients with primary dupuytren's contracture: a prospective, randomized, controlled trial. Plast Reconstr Surg 2016;137(6): 1800–12.

Complications of Treatment for Dupuytren Disease

Kyle R. Eberlin, MD[a],
Chaitanya S. Mudgal, MD, MS(Orth), MCh(Orth)[b],*

KEYWORDS

- Dupuytren • Contracture • Complication • Nerve injury • Wound healing

KEY POINTS

- Many treatment options exist for Dupuytren contracture, including collagenase injection, fasciotomy, and fasciectomy; each has its own complication profile.
- Complications should be recognized: digital nerve and arterial injuries should be addressed immediately, whereas wound-healing complications are often treated nonoperatively.
- A thorough preoperative discussion is imperative to optimize the risk/benefit tolerance before intervention.
- In severe, long-standing contractures, complete correction may not only be impossible but may also be imprudent. It is vital that patients be counseled suitably about this via a thorough preoperative discussion.

INTRODUCTION

Dupuytren contracture is a progressive disorder involving collagen within the palmar fascia of the hand. It is most often attributed to the French anatomist and military surgeon Baron Guillaume Dupuytren from his description in 1831,[1] and occurs primarily in individuals of Northern European descent.[2,3] It is a condition of great interest to hand surgeons, as it is one of the few genetically associated hand conditions with an onset in adulthood. The precise etiology is still largely unknown.

There are multiple patterns of disease progression; some patients have gradual development of the characteristic nodules and cords of the disease but do not progress to severe contracture, whereas others develop a rapidly progressive disease that causes significant functional impairment. Although the patterns and progression of Dupuytren contracture have been studied,[4] it is often difficult to predict the natural history for an individual patient.

Intervention is traditionally considered for patients with functional impairment and contractures of the metacarpophalangeal (MCP) joint more than 30° or any degree of proximal interphalangeal (PIP) joint contracture.[5,6] Options for treatment are numerous and include percutaneous and open fasciotomy,[7–9] injection of collagenase *Clostridium* histolyticum,[10–12] radiation therapy,[13] and subtotal or complete palmar fasciectomy.[14–17] Each treatment option has utility and may be used for specific patients depending on their degree of contracture and the functional requirements for treatment.

Disclosure Statement: Neither author has a financial interest or relationship in anything related to this article.
[a] MGH Hand Surgery Fellowship, Harvard Plastic Surgery Residency Program, Massachusetts General Hospital, Harvard Medical School, 55 Fruit Street, Boston, MA 02114, USA; [b] Hand Surgery Service, Department of Orthopaedics, Yawkey Center, Massachusetts General Hospital, Harvard Medical School, 55 Fruit Street, Boston, MA 02114, USA
* Corresponding author.
E-mail address: cmudgal@mgh.harvard.edu

Dupuytren contracture often has minimal functional impairment until it limits sufficient extension of the digits and prohibits prehension. For this reason, the objective criteria used when deciding about intervention may vary significantly between surgeons and between patients. There exists a paradox regarding surgical intervention for Dupuytren contracture: surgeons and patients desire to avoid intervention for as long as possible, but durable correction becomes increasingly difficult with advanced disease and fixed contractures. Given the potential complications of intervention, one must thoughtfully consider both the risks and benefits before deciding about intervention.

A thorough preoperative examination is critical, including specific measurements of both active and passive ranges of motion of the MCP, proximal interphalangeal (PIP), and distal interphalangeal (DIP) joints. A precise sensory examination is also recommended to determine baseline sensibility of the affected digits. In long-standing and/or severe PIP contractures, radiographs are recommended to evaluate the articular surfaces of the involved joints. Radiographic findings of degenerative changes must be communicated with the patient, because they have a bearing on the degree and durability of final correction.

COMPLICATIONS OF TREATMENT

There are many potential complications in the treatment of Dupuytren contracture. The nature of these complications depends on many factors, including the degree of contracture, rapidity of development, duration of disease, involvement of the PIP joint, and the intervention chosen.[18]

Contracture Recurrence

Contracture recurrence is nearly inevitable following treatment for Dupuytren disease, particularly when patients are followed carefully over an extended period of time. This general category of complication includes both disease and contracture recurrence, which often coexist but may be independent. Disease recurrence involves return of fascial pathology, which may involve increasing flexion of the digit; contracture recurrence specifically entails progression of MCP or PIP joint contracture independent of recurrent fascial disease.

As most patients will develop some degree of recurrence, an objective definition of this complication is essential. Depending on the definition, the recurrence rates after treatment may vary between 0% and 100%,[11,19,20] which underscores the importance of a uniform definition when describing the rate of recurrence. Even within a single patient cohort, recurrence rates after treatment can vary widely, from 2% to 86%, depending on the exact definition used.[21] With a lack of overall consensus about the precise definition of recurrence, it is difficult to accurately compare results between different studies. A clear definition of recurrence is needed.[22]

For this reason, in 2017 Kan and colleagues[23] used expert consensus and the Delphi method[24] (at least 70% agreement among experts) to determine the definition for recurrence. In this article, the investigators agreed that recurrence should be defined as "more than 20° of contracture recurrence in any treated joint at 1 year posttreatment compared with 6 weeks posttreatment." Although imperfect, this may be the best definition to date, and may be used for future comparative studies (**Fig. 1**).

Hindocha and colleagues[25] described 5 risk factors for Dupuytren recurrence after treatment: family history, bilateral disease, ectopic lesions, male sex, and age of onset less than 50 years. Contracture recurrence may be evident within 6 months after surgery.[26] Although comparative studies are still being performed, there appears

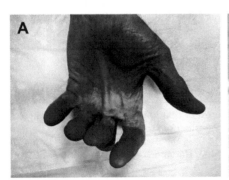
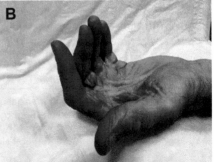

Fig. 1. (*A*, *B*) A 68-year-old man demonstrating recurrence 13 years after open fasciectomy and 4 years after collagenase injection to the ulnar 3 digits of the left hand. Complete correction was achieved after both procedures. (*Courtesy of* C. Mudgal, MD, Boston, MA.)

to be a lower risk of recurrence with open fasciec-tomy versus percutaneous fasciotomy,[20] and a lower rate with open surgery versus collagenase treatment.[27] As fasciectomy is a more intensive intervention, the choice of optimal treatment depends on many factors.

Regardless of the intervention performed, contracture recurrence is an expected sequela of Dupuytren treatment, although the time frame and severity of recurrence vary between patients. Secondary treatment of disease recurrence may involve any of the described treatment modalities, although salvage fasciectomy after initial treatment with collagenase may be more difficult than primary surgery.[28]

Digital Nerve Injury and Postoperative Neurapraxia

Digital nerve injury is an unfortunate complication of treatment for Dupuytren contracture. Nerve symptoms following Dupuytren surgery generally fall into 1 of 2 categories: neurapraxia and nerve transection.

Postoperative numbness and paresthesias in the absence of surgical nerve injury (ie, neurapraxia) are common and can occur in up to 46% of patients undergoing fasciectomy.[29] In the authors' experience, nearly all patients undergoing fasciectomy experience, at minimum, peri-incisional numbness or distal paresthesias in the immediate postoperative period, if questioned specifically about these symptoms. Neurapraxia ultimately resolves without intervention within 2 to 3 months, although persistent numbness and/or a Tinel sign after this period should alert the surgeon about the potential presence of a nerve injury. Neuropathic pain is an additional sign of nerve injury and may indicate the presence of a symptomatic neuroma (**Fig. 2**).

Digital nerve transection is a feared and unfortunate complication of open surgery for Dupuytren contracture. Injury to a digital nerve is relatively uncommon and occurs in fewer than 10% of patients undergoing operative intervention, but is an iatrogenic and avoidable complication of surgery. Multiple prior series have reported complication rates for digital nerve injuries during fasciectomy: 7.7% by Tubiana and colleagues,[30] 5.2% by Hoet and colleagues,[31] 7.8% by Sennwald,[32] 1.9% by Foucher and colleagues,[33] and 2.0% by Bulstrode and colleagues.[34] Needle fasciotomy appears to confer a lower risk of digital nerve injury compared with fasciectomy, ranging from 1% to 4%.[8,35,36] If digital nerve injury occurs intraoperatively, it warrants immediate operative repair and this is usually undertaken with the operating microscope.

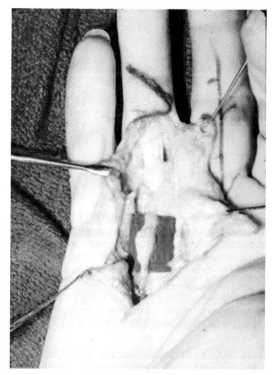

Fig. 2. Persistent pain and numbness after fasciectomy. Exploration revealed a transected nerve with a neuroma-in-continuity. (*Courtesy of* P. Stern, MD, Cincinnati, OH.)

To avoid inadvertent nerve injury during Dupuytren surgery, it is imperative to understand the anatomic displacement of the neurovascular structures that can occur with development of Dupuytren cords, particularly abductor digiti minimi cords, lateral cords, and spiral cords. It is advisable to identify the neurovascular structures proximally and trace them distally (or vice versa) to avoid nerve injury during surgery. Dissection superficial to the fibers of Skoog (the mid-palmar transverse fascial bands) is usually safe, because the neurovascular structures remain deep to these fibers. However, distal to the fibers of Skoog, the neurovascular bundle can get displaced centrally, proximally, and superficially, typically due to a spiral cord. Meticulous dissection in this area is vital to avoid injury to the neurovascular bundles.

In the presence of an abductor digiti minimi cord, special care with dissection of the ulnar digital nerve of the small finger is required. This nerve is particularly prone to injury on the deep surface of the cord, as well as at ulnar edge of the PIP flexion crease (**Fig. 3**).

Flexor Tendon Injury/Rupture

Flexor tendon injury or rupture is another uncommon but devastating complication of Dupuytren

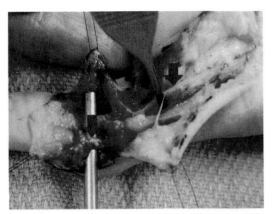

Fig. 3. The unique anatomic features of the ulnar digital nerve of the small finger in the setting of an abductor digiti minimi cord, which can make the nerve vulnerable to iatrogenic injury. The metallic instruments show the nerve displaced proximally and radially and then traveling deep to the cord to emerge at the ulnar edge of the PIP flexion crease (*blue arrows* indicate proximal and distal nerve). (*Courtesy of* C. Mudgal, MD, Boston, MA.)

treatment. Pathophysiologically, Dupuytren disease lies within the palmar fascia, superficial to and distinct from the flexor tendons. The flexor tendons, however, can be injured in an attempt to resect or create discontinuity in the cords (ie, fasciotomy) as both cords and flexor tendons become more taut with digital extension.

Flexor tendon injury is more common following the "less invasive" treatments in which the flexor tendons are not directly visualized. Rates of tendon injury during percutaneous needle fasciotomy have been reported as 0.05%,[35] and slightly higher with collagenase *Clostridium* histolyticum (Xiaflex) treatment, 0.27%, particularly in the small finger.[37] If a flexor tendon is injured during percutaneous needle fasciotomy, it may be amenable to primary tendon repair, but rupture after collagenase *Clostridium* histolyticum tendon often necessitates 2-stage tendon reconstruction.

To avoid flexor tendon injury during needle fasciotomy, it is important to perform gentle excursion of the flexor tendon periodically during the procedure to ensure that the needle is not stuck within the flexor tendon or in the tendon sheath.[38] During collagenase injection, it is recommended to inject not more than 4 mm distal to the palmar digital crease, and to inject in a coronal plane (horizontally) in this region, so as not to inject within the substance of the tendon.[37]

Delayed Wound Healing and Skin Necrosis

Delayed wound healing, defined as skin tears following digital manipulation or dehiscence

following wound closure, is a common complication after open palmar fasciectomy, percutaneous needle fasciotomy, and collagenase injection. After fasciectomy, poor wound healing can occur because of marginal or diminished perfusion of the skin flaps. Skin tears after needle fasciotomy or collagenase injection are often related to digital extension without accommodation of the skin, although most of these heal within 4 weeks.

In a systematic review, wound-healing complications were found in 22.9% (range 0%–86%) of patients undergoing fasciectomy, although this included varying degrees of skin necrosis and dehiscence.[39] Most of the time, wound complications after fasciectomy can be managed nonoperatively and eventually heal (**Fig. 4**). Like most complications related to Dupuytren treatment, the risk of wound-healing complications appears to be higher in those undergoing secondary surgery. In one study of patients undergoing repeat fasciectomy, delayed healing was found in 42.9% of patients, but all healed completely within 4 weeks.[40]

Skin fissures/tears are common in patients undergoing percutaneous fasciotomy, with occurrences in up to 50% of patients.[9,35,41] This complication may be at least partially avoidable with some technical modifications to the procedure, such as tangential dissection to release the skin from the underlying cord before manipulation into extension.[38] Such skin tears are also common in patients receiving collagenase, particularly when the MCP joint has greater than a 50° contracture[37,41] (**Fig. 5**). It is important to discuss this possibility with patients before the procedure, as this can be disconcerting if they are unaware of this risk. In the authors' practice, skin tears are almost always managed nonoperatively with a moist dressing using bacitracin and Xeroform, changed 2 or 3 times daily. Range of motion and formal hand therapy continue during the phase of soft tissue healing.

Dysvascular Digit/Arterial Injury

Perhaps the most feared complication of Dupuytren surgery is digital arterial injury and subsequent necrosis of the digit. In a systematic review, digital arterial injury was reported in 2% of patients undergoing fasciectomy,[39] which is similar to the incidence of digital nerve injury (and not surprising given their proximate anatomic location). It also has been reported after collagenase treatment.[42]

As there is significant redundancy in digital perfusion, injury to the digital vessels infrequently results in critical digital ischemia, as collateral perfusion can usually maintain viability of the digit.

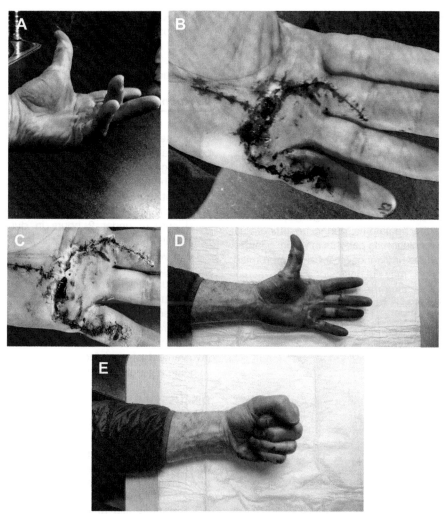

Fig. 4. (*A*) Preoperative appearance in a 52-year-old man with Dupuytren disease. After open fasciectomy, (*B*) wound breakdown was noted on the fifth day, and (*C*) advancing wound edge separation noted on the 12th day after surgery. The wound was managed using local wound care and moist dressing changes. (*D, E*) Final appearance and function 3 months after surgery. (*Courtesy of* C. Mudgal, MD, Boston, MA.)

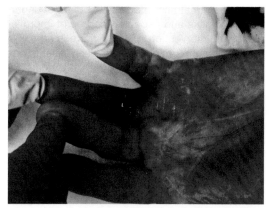

Fig. 5. Skin tear after injection of collagenase. The tear healed uneventfully with local wound care. (*Courtesy of* P. Blazar, MD, Boston, MA.)

This must not be taken for granted, however, as digit-threatening ischemia may occur; emergent microsurgical revascularization has been reported for salvage in these cases.[43] It is the authors' policy to add the possibility of digital ischemia and/or digital neurovascular injury to the consent form and to discuss this specifically with patients before surgery.

Most often, apparent digital ischemia in the operating room following fasciectomy is related to vasospasm rather than arterial transection. Treatment consists of warming the digit, antispasm agents such as papaverine or lidocaine, and/or flexing the digit to relieve undue tension on the vessel. The overall duration of these maneuvers should be 10 minutes at minimum, which will usually result in a pink, warm digit with appropriate capillary refill. If the digit remains ischemic, further investigation and exploration of the digital vessels should be undertaken and revascularization performed, if required.

Hematoma

Hematoma is most commonly seen after open fasciectomy, occurring in approximately 2% of cases.[39] In most circumstances, these tend to occur if meticulous attention has not been paid to hemostasis during the procedure, and when closure is performed before deflation of the tourniquet. If diagnosed early in the postoperative course, removal of a few strategic sutures and expressing the hematoma during an office visit will lead to resolution. In patients in whom a larger hematoma goes undiagnosed, it can compromise flap viability and may not only necessitate evacuation in the operating room, but may also lead to compromise of skin flaps (**Fig. 6**).

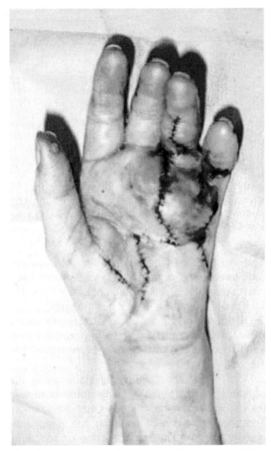

Fig. 6. Hematoma after open fasciectomy. After removal of a few sutures, hematoma was expressed with uneventful recovery. (*Courtesy of* P. Stern, MD, Cincinnati, OH.)

Collagenase injection is often associated with ecchymosis and hemorrhagic blisters at the site(s) of injection, but rarely results in a true hematoma. These findings do not require additional intervention.[10]

Infection

Infection is an uncommon complication that may occur after open fasciectomy; it is rarely seen after collagenase injection. It is usually associated with some degree of flap necrosis and tends to be superficial. Although there have been no formal studies investigating the efficacy of antibiotic prophylaxis specifically for Dupuytren surgery, most elective hand surgery under 2 hours in duration does not require the use of prophylactic antibiotics.[44]

Local wound care and oral antibiotics, targeting gram-positive organisms, typically lead to resolution of superficial infections. Formal irrigation and debridement are rarely required, but should be performed when the wound does not respond to local care or when there is concern for deep sepsis. In cases requiring operative debridement, involvement of an infectious disease consultant to guide antibiotic treatment is recommended.

DISCUSSION

Complications following intervention for Dupuytren contracture vary in frequency, severity, and impact. Primary prevention of these complications may be possible with meticulous surgical planning and careful operative technique.

Patient education is paramount to managing the risk/benefit profile of intervention and expectations for surgery. If Dupuytren disease is present, but has minimal functional impact, it is usually preferable to pursue clinical observation and nonoperative management. If the disease progresses, patients and surgeons may choose from the various treatment modalities, but must understand the risks and expected degree of improvement with intervention. Usually, there is no single best treatment option for a given patient; one must take into account the patient's goals for treatment, functional requirements, understanding of time frame for recovery, and tolerance for complications. Shared decision making has a significant role in the choice of treatment for Dupuytren contracture and may lead to improved outcomes with greater patient satisfaction.[45–47]

To this end, it is our practice to evaluate patients more than once before deciding about the timing and type of intervention. Patients should be given sufficient information to make an informed decision about the treatment choices, particularly with regard to potential complications.

Some of the aforementioned complications resulting from Dupuytren treatment mandate immediate assessment and intervention (such as a digital nerve injury), whereas others are optimally addressed by providing observation and reassurance (such as delayed wound healing). It is incumbent on the surgeon to understand all possible outcomes and to provide the optimal treatment for complications if they arise.

Not surprisingly, patients with more severe Dupuytren contracture appear to have more frequent complications than those with less severe pathology,[3] particularly if there is a PIP contracture greater than 60°.[34] This finding is likely secondary to the invasiveness of intervention, with greater requirement for soft tissue dissection, joint release, and so forth. Certain complications are significantly more common in patients undergoing treatment for recurrence; digital nerve and arterial injuries appear to be approximately 10-fold more common during surgery for recurrent disease.[39]

Future studies and potential interventions may be directed, in a preventive way, at the yet-determined causal agent of Dupuytren disease. If the disease process could be halted before the development of clinically apparent disease and the resultant contractures, this would potentially reduce or prevent the need for surgical intervention.

REFERENCES

1. Dupuytren G. Permanent retraction of the fingers, produced by an affection of the palmar fascia. Lancet 1834;2:222–5.
2. Early PF. Population studies in Dupuytren's contracture. J Bone Joint Surg Am 1962;44:602–13.
3. Loos B, Puschkin V, Horch RE. 50 years experience with Dupuytren's contracture in the Erlangen University Hospital–a retrospective analysis of 2919 operated hands from 1956 to 2006. BMC Musculoskelet Disord 2007;8:60.
4. Mikkelsen OA. Dupuytren's disease–a study of the pattern of distribution and stage of contracture in the hand. Hand 1976;8(3):265–71.
5. Rayan GM. Dupuytren disease: anatomy, pathology, presentation, and treatment. J Bone Joint Surg Am 2007;89(1):189–98.
6. Smith AC. Diagnosis and indications for surgical treatment. Hand Clin 1991;7(4):635–42 [discussion: 643].
7. Citron N, Hearnden A. Skin tension in the aetiology of Dupuytren's disease; a prospective trial. J Hand Surg Br 2003;28(6):528–30.
8. Foucher G, Medina J, Navarro R. Percutaneous needle aponeurotomy: complications and results. J Hand Surg Br 2003;28(5):427–31.
9. van Rijssen AL, Gerbrandy FS, Ter Linden H, et al. A comparison of the direct outcomes of percutaneous needle fasciotomy and limited fasciectomy for Dupuytren's disease: a 6-week follow-up study. J Hand Surg 2006;31(5):717–25.
10. Hurst LC, Badalamente MA, Hentz VR, et al. Injectable collagenase Clostridium histolyticum for Dupuytren's contracture. N Engl J Med 2009;361(10):968–79.
11. Gilpin D, Coleman S, Hall S, et al. Injectable collagenase Clostridium histolyticum: a new nonsurgical treatment for Dupuytren's disease. J Hand Surg 2010;35(12):2027–38.e1.
12. Starkweather KD, Lattuga S, Hurst LC, et al. Collagenase in the treatment of Dupuytren's disease: an in vitro study. J Hand Surg 1996;21(3):490–5.
13. Keilholz L, Seegenschmiedt MH, Sauer R. Radiotherapy for prevention of disease progression in early-stage Dupuytren's contracture: initial and long-term results. Int J Radiat Oncol Biol Phys 1996;36(4):891–7.
14. Coert JH, Nerin JP, Meek MF. Results of partial fasciectomy for Dupuytren disease in 261 consecutive patients. Ann Plast Surg 2006;57(1):13–7.
15. Shaw RB Jr, Chong AK, Zhang A, et al. Dupuytren's disease: history, diagnosis, and treatment. Plast Reconstr Surg 2007;120(3):44e–54e.
16. Desai SS, Hentz VR. The treatment of Dupuytren disease. J Hand Surg 2011;36(5):936–42.
17. Bayat A, McGrouther DA. Management of Dupuytren's disease–clear advice for an elusive condition. Ann R Coll Surg Engl 2006;88(1):3–8.
18. Cheung K, Walley KC, Rozental TD. Management of complications of Dupuytren contracture. Hand Clin 2015;31(2):345–54.
19. Brotherston TM, Balakrishnan C, Milner RH, et al. Long term follow-up of dermofasciectomy for Dupuytren's contracture. Br J Plast Surg 1994;47(6):440–3.
20. van Rijssen AL, ter Linden H, Werker PM. Five-year results of a randomized clinical trial on treatment in Dupuytren's disease: percutaneous needle fasciotomy versus limited fasciectomy. Plast Reconstr Surg 2012;129(2):469–77.
21. Kan HJ, Verrijp FW, Huisstede BM, et al. The consequences of different definitions for recurrence of Dupuytren's disease. J Plast Reconstr Aesthet Surg 2013;66(1):95–103.
22. Werker PM, Pess GM, van Rijssen AL, et al. Correction of contracture and recurrence rates of Dupuytren contracture following invasive treatment: the importance of clear definitions. J Hand Surg 2012;37(10):2095–105.e7.
23. Kan HJ, Verrijp FW, Hovius SER, et al. Recurrence of Dupuytren's contracture: a consensus-based definition. PLoS One 2017;12(5):e0164849.

24. Hasson F, Keeney S, McKenna H. Research guidelines for the Delphi survey technique. J Adv Nurs 2000;32(4):1008–15.

25. Hindocha S, Stanley JK, Watson S, et al. Dupuytren's diathesis revisited: evaluation of prognostic indicators for risk of disease recurrence. J Hand Surg 2006;31(10):1626–34.

26. Dias JJ, Singh HP, Ullah A, et al. Patterns of recontracture after surgical correction of Dupuytren disease. J Hand Surg 2013;38(10):1987–93.

27. Peimer CA, Blazar P, Coleman S, et al. Dupuytren contracture recurrence following treatment with collagenase clostridium histolyticum (CORDLESS study): 3-year data. J Hand Surg 2013;38(1):12–22.

28. Eberlin KR, Kobraei EM, Nyame TT, et al. Salvage palmar fasciectomy after initial treatment with collagenase clostridium histolyticum. Plast Reconstr Surg 2015;135(6):1000e–6e.

29. Ullah AS, Dias JJ, Bhowal B. Does a 'firebreak' full-thickness skin graft prevent recurrence after surgery for Dupuytren's contracture? A prospective, randomised trial. J Bone Joint Surg Br 2009;91(3):374–8.

30. Tubiana R, Thomine JM, Brown S. Complications in surgery of Dupuytren's contracture. Plast Reconstr Surg 1967;39(6):603–12.

31. Hoet F, Boxho J, Decoster E, et al. Dupuytren's disease. Review of 326 surgically treated patients. Ann Chir Main 1988;7(3):251–5 [in French].

32. Sennwald GR. Fasciectomy for treatment of Dupuytren's disease and early complications. J Hand Surg 1990;15(5):755–61.

33. Foucher G, Cornil C, Lenoble E, et al. A modified open palm technique for Dupuytren's disease. Short and long term results in 54 patients. Int Orthop 1995;19(5):285–8.

34. Bulstrode NW, Jemec B, Smith PJ. The complications of Dupuytren's contracture surgery. J Hand Surg 2005;30(5):1021–5.

35. Beaudreuil J, Lellouche H, Orcel P, et al. Needle aponeurotomy in Dupuytren's disease. Joint Bone Spine 2012;79(1):13–6.

36. Pess GM, Pess RM, Pess RA. Results of needle aponeurotomy for Dupuytren contracture in over 1,000 fingers. J Hand Surg 2012;37(4):651–6.

37. Hentz VR, Watt AJ, Desai SS, et al. Advances in the management of Dupuytren disease: collagenase. Hand Clin 2012;28(4):551–63.

38. Eaton C. Percutaneous fasciotomy for Dupuytren's contracture. J Hand Surg 2011;36(5):910–5.

39. Denkler K. Surgical complications associated with fasciectomy for Dupuytren's disease: a 20-year review of the English literature. Eplasty 2010;10:e15.

40. Konneker S, Broelsch GF, Krezdorn N, et al. Multiple recurrences in aggressive forms of Dupuytren's disease—can patients benefit from repeated selective fasciectomy? Plast Reconstr Surg Glob Open 2017;5(2):e1247.

41. Nydick JA, Olliff BW, Garcia MJ, et al. A comparison of percutaneous needle fasciotomy and collagenase injection for Dupuytren disease. J Hand Surg 2013;38(12):2377–80.

42. Spiers JD, Ullah A, Dias JJ. Vascular complication after collagenase injection and manipulation for Dupuytren's contracture. J Hand Surg Eur Vol 2014;39(5):554–6.

43. Jones NF, Huang JI. Emergency microsurgical revascularization for critical ischemia during surgery for Dupuytren's contracture: a case report. J Hand Surg 2001;26(6):1125–8.

44. Eberlin KR, Ring D. Infection after hand surgery. Hand Clin 2015;31(2):355–60.

45. Barry MJ, Edgman-Levitan S. Shared decision making–pinnacle of patient-centered care. N Engl J Med 2012;366(9):780–1.

46. Bot AG, Bossen JK, Herndon JH, et al. Informed shared decision-making and patient satisfaction. Psychosomatics 2014;55(6):586–94.

47. Vranceanu AM, Cooper C, Ring D. Integrating patient values into evidence-based practice: effective communication for shared decision-making. Hand Clin 2009;25(1):83–96, vii.

The Role of Hand Therapy in Dupuytren Disease

Christina Turesson, ROT, PhD[a,b,*]

KEYWORDS

- Dupuytren disease • Edema • Exercise • Hand therapy • Orthoses • Patient education • Scar

KEY POINTS

- Hand therapy as preventive treatment of Dupuytren disease (DD) is uncommon, with limited evidence to support its usefulness.
- Before corrective treatment, a hand therapist can perform an assessment of hand function and daily activities to assist in a systematic evaluation of outcomes after treatment.
- After corrective treatment, hand therapy is tailored to each patient's needs and consists of interventions, such as orthoses, exercise, edema control, and pain or scar management.
- Orthoses are usually part of the hand therapy protocol after corrective procedures for DD despite lack of strong evidence to support this intervention.
- It is recommended to provide orthoses based on individual patient needs instead of providing them routinely to every patient.

INTRODUCTION

The overall aims of hand therapy are to prevent, restore, and reverse the progression of upper limb pathologies to enhance an individual's ability to execute tasks and participate in daily life.[1,2] For patients with Dupuytren disease (DD), hand therapy also aims to maintain the achieved gains in finger extension and minimize the negative effects of treatment.[3–5] To achieve these goals, a hand therapist commonly uses multiple treatment modalities, such as orthoses, active exercises, edema control, scar management, and patient education, depending on a patient's needs.[6]

HAND THERAPY AS PREVENTIVE TREATMENT

Patients with DD usually seek medical care when hand function is negatively affected, and this state is interfering with daily activities.[7] It is uncommon in clinical practice, however, that patients are referred to a hand therapist for preventive treatment, and evidence to support its use in early DD is limited. In previous research, different techniques, such as orthoses, frictional massage, or heat treatment with joint stretching, have been examined for the treatment of patients with palmar nodule or limited or no finger contractures. Despite the tendency for improved digital joint extension using these techniques, alone or in combination, a systematic review has concluded there is insufficient evidence of their efficacy.[8] The rationales for these treatment techniques were to promote tissue remodeling by applying low-load tension through orthoses or tissue mobilization[9,10] and to reduce the fibrous adhesions using cross-frictional massage.[11]

The use of orthotic devices for preventive treatment of DD has been further investigated in a recently published pilot randomized controlled trial

Disclosure Statement: The author reports no declarations of interest.
[a] Department of Hand Surgery, Plastic Surgery and Burns, Linköping University Hospital, Linköping University, Linköping 581 85, Sweden; [b] Department of Social and Welfare Studies, Linköping University, Kungsgatan 40, Norrköping 60174, Sweden
* Department of Hand Surgery, Plastic Surgery and Burns, Linköping University Hospital, Linköping 581 85, Sweden.
E-mail address: christina.turesson@regionostergotland.se

Hand Clin 34 (2018) 395–401
https://doi.org/10.1016/j.hcl.2018.03.008

(RCT). The study investigated 2 orthotic devices as preventive treatment in patients with previously untreated DD or postoperative recurrent disease. Patients were randomized into 2 groups and were treated with different orthoses (tension or compression) that were to be used 20 hours a day for 3 months. Both groups improved from baseline average total extension deficits of 53° and 65° to 32° and 46°, respectively, but there were no statistically significant differences between the groups. In conclusion, the study showed that the extension deficit can be influenced with a tension or compression orthotic device used for many hours a day. The long-term results of using an orthotic device as a preventive or delaying strategy, however, need to be investigated further.[12]

HAND THERAPY BEFORE CORRECTIVE TREATMENT

Although the finger contractures can be corrected, this does not cure DD and the disease is likely to recur or extend after treatment.[13,14] Preoperatively, a hand therapist can contribute an assessment of physical measures of hand function as well as collecting patient-reported outcomes to be used for short-term and long-term follow-up. Assessments of physical function should include measures of finger joint range of motion, grip strength, sensibility, and pain.[15,16] Pain has not commonly been associated with DD, but the findings of Rodrigues and colleagues[16] showed that 15% of the patients with DD (n = 110) experienced pain as a functional problem. Patient-reported outcomes targeting both function and activity should also be included in the preoperative assessment. In previous research, the Disabilities of the Arm, Shoulder and Hand (DASH) questionnaire has been the most frequently used patient-reported outcome instrument.[15] Disease-specific questionnaires also exist, such as the Unité Rhumatologique des Affections de la Main (URAM) scale[17,18] or the Southampton Dupuytren's Scoring scheme.[19] Questions have been raised concerning whether DASH is an appropriate instrument to use in patients with DD due to ceiling effects or if interpretation of minimal important change is applicable to these patients.[20–23] The URAM scale has shown acceptable responsiveness[23] but has been criticized for failing to capture common problems among patients with DD, such as difficulty with putting on a glove or putting a hand in a pocket.[16] Because patients with DD experience a wide range of problems in their daily lives, an individualized approach to patient-reported outcomes may be useful. For a pragmatic and patient-centered approach, patients can be asked to define tasks that are difficult to perform and rate their performance before and after treatment.[24] Furthermore, safety and social issues of hand function, that is, the need to take special precautions due to hand function or the avoidance of using the hand in social contexts, should also be included in patient-reported outcomes because these play an important part in patients' rating of functioning.[25]

HAND THERAPY AFTER CORRECTIVE TREATMENT

Hand therapy after corrective treatment consists of different modalities, such as orthoses, active exercises, edema control, scar management, and patient education. The extent of intervention depends on the corrective procedure and the phases of tissue healing.[4] Because hand therapy is usually provided and evaluated in combination with surgery or other corrective treatment,[3,26–31] there is evidence to support hand therapy for patients with DD given in this combination. Research regarding the benefits of hand therapy alone for patients with DD is, however, lacking. Herweijer and colleagues[32] investigated the difference in outcomes after surgery between patients receiving hand therapy or not by comparing patients correctly referred for postoperative hand therapy compared with those incorrectly not referred for hand therapy. The hand therapy protocol used in the study consisted of static orthoses, range-of-motion exercises, edema reduction, and silicone dressing to limit scar hypertrophy. Orthoses were initially used for 24 hours a day, then gradually removed during day-time after the wound was healed and continued at night-time for 6 months. No statistical significant differences were found between the groups, although the group receiving hand therapy had a tendency for greater improvement in joint mobility. The study had several limitations, including small sample size, differences between the groups regarding severity of the disease, and no randomization. These limitations make it difficult to draw definitive conclusions about the efficacy of a postoperative hand therapy protocol.

Orthoses

Orthoses have historically been used after hand surgery and trauma as a way to apply a low-load prolonged stretch to promote soft tissue remodeling.[33] For patients with DD, orthoses have commonly been used in hand therapy to maintain the achieved gains in finger extension. The orthotic intervention usually starts after reduction of dressings, and the orthosis can initially be worn 24 hours a day during the first week, and this gradually continues to nighttime use to enable functional use of the hand. Follow-up of patients for 1 year after surgery for DD has shown that many patients (37%, n = 84) still use the orthosis 6 months after surgery.[31]

Research regarding orthoses has investigated their effect on range of motion and self-reported function, scarring, and flare reactions (reactive erythema, stiffness, and edema). The effect on range of motion has been investigated for both dynamic and static orthoses, and the evidence supporting this intervention is weak.[34,35] For dynamic extension orthoses, the evidence is inconclusive and of low level, showing a positive effect on severe proximal interphalangeal (PIP) joint contractures[36] but no effect on the natural course of the disease.[37] Three different RCT studies have investigated the effect of static postoperative orthoses for patients with DD.[38–40] All the studies showed the same result: orthoses in combination with hand therapy were no better than hand therapy alone in minimizing postoperative extension deficit of the finger joints. It is also unclear whether the use of orthoses plays a part in impaired finger flexion postoperatively.[31,35] Two studies investigated the position of the fingers in the orthosis and the effect of tension applied to the metacarpophalangeal (MCP) joints. Both studies showed that a nontension approach, placing the MCP joints in slight flexion, was better than placing extension forces to the MCP joints during wound healing. The nontension approach led to less scar formation and fewer flare reactions.[41,42]

Orthoses have also been used after treatment with needle aponeurotomy[43,44] and after collagenase Clostridium histolyticum (CCH) injection.[45] Still, the evidence for the use of orthoses is of low level, that is, case study[43] or retrospective study,[44] and inconclusive regarding their effect. Scherman and colleagues[45] compared outcomes in patients with predominantly MCP joint involvement treated with needle fasciotomy or collagenase injection at 2 different centers. Only 1 center provided patients with a night extension orthosis for 3 months in combination with the corrective procedure, giving the opportunity to also compare differences in outcome based on the use of orthoses. No differences were found between the groups. The sample size was small, however, and no power calculation was performed for this comparison.

The need for hand therapy after CCH injection has been suggested to be limited to orthotic intervention only.[46] The initial CORD 1 (the Collagenase Option for Reduction of Dupuytren's, a phase 3 clinical trial) protocol included 4 months of nighttime use of an orthosis,[47] and many recent studies have continued with this recommendation.[48–52] The severity of contracture of affected joints has to be taken into consideration, however, when discussing the need for hand therapy after CCH injection. It has been shown that a specific postinjection orthotic intervention protocol, in combination with targeted exercises, has a positive effect on severe PIP joint contractures 4 weeks after treatment with injection.[53] Because the study design included no control group; however, further research is needed to establish evidence for the effect of postinjection orthosis beyond 4 weeks.

It has been recommended to provide orthoses primarily to patients who lose finger joint extension rapidly in the early postoperative period, instead of providing it routinely to every patient.[38,39,54] A European expert group has recommended orthotic intervention for severe cases, after open procedures, or for patients with large preoperative contractures of the PIP joint.[55]

Exercise

An important part of hand therapy is to restore full finger joint range of motion. DD leads to prolonged immobilization of finger joints, which in turn leads to shortening of joint structures, for example, joint capsules, ligaments, fascia, and so forth. These preexisting changes are, together with postoperative issues, a challenge to address.[56] Therefore, exercise programs are an important part of hand therapy to maximize functional use of the hand and to prevent joint stiffness.[57] Range-of-motion exercises are usually included in postoperative hand therapy after corrective procedures for DD.[24,31,32,40,44,53,58] Thus, there is evidence for range-of-motion exercise as part of a hand therapy protocol for these patients. Michlovitz and colleagues[59] concluded that there is moderate evidence for the use of exercise for managing joint contractures in the upper limbs. Few studies have investigated finger joint contractures specifically, however, and the best exercise intensity or frequency is unclear. Therefore, to choose the most appropriate quantity of treatment or exercise for a given situation, a hand therapist needs understanding of the soft tissue response to stress. Generally, active motion provides a lower level of load than passive range of motion. Hence, active motion is started as early as possible in the inflammatory and early fibroblastic stages of tissue healing, whereas passive range-of-motion or resistance exercises can be introduced in a later stage of tissue healing.[57,60] For patients with DD, special attention should be given to the PIP joint because outcomes after treatment are usually better for the MCP than for the PIP joint,[51,61,62] and the PIP joint needs a longer time for recovery after surgical intervention.[31] Gentle composite finger flexion exercise usually starts during the first week after surgery and progresses during weeks 2 and 3—as the wounds are healing—to include isolated tendon gliding, hook, and full fist. Aggressive exercise should be avoided to minimize complications.[63]

Several factors, for example, infection, delayed wound healing, and complex regional pain syndrome, can contribute to prolonged digital stiffness and poor hand function. In a small case series, Midgley[56] investigated a casting motion to mobilize stiffness (CMMS) technique for 4 patients with DD suffering from persistent digital stiffness and a poor pattern of motion in the operated hand. The CMMS technique includes a nonremovable plaster of Paris cast that immobilizes proximal joints in an ideal position and limits distal joint movement within a desired direction and range. This cast can be maintained for a prolonged period of time to encourage active motion at the desired joints.[64] The 4 patients in this study were treated with a cast blocking MCP joint extension but allowing interphalangeal joint flexion to elongate the intrinsic muscles. The cast was worn on average for 11 weeks, and the patients performed exercises in the cast and used the casted hand in functional activities. The results showed a positive response with improved finger flexion and pattern of motion without compromising the digital extension gained during surgery.[56] Further research is needed, however, to provide conclusive evidence for the use of the CMMS technique in patients with DD suffering from persistent joint stiffness.

Other Treatment Modalities

Hand therapy after corrective treatment can also involve other treatment modalities that can be applied depending on an individual patient's specific problems. Complications after surgery for DD include, among others, edema, scar hypertrophy, and flare reactions.[61,65] Thus, swelling, scarring, or pain may need to be addressed in hand therapy. As in all hand conditions treated with surgery, edema control is crucial; examples of interventions include elevation, active motion, and/or pressure garments.[66] Intervention directed toward swelling, that is, compression gloves or finger wrapping, can be needed by 30% of the patients during the first 3 months after fasciectomy for DD, whereas 12% may need intervention for scar issues.[31] Scar management can consist of massage, desensitization, tape, or occlusive materials, such as silicone gel sheets.[63] Massage

has an established role in hand therapy and is used to soften tissue and increase or maintain functional mobility.[55,67] Pain can be addressed with transcutaneous electrical nerve stimulation or acupuncture.[31]

Patient Education and Participation

An important part of clinical practice is to encourage patients to be actively involved in the postoperative rehabilitation, because many of the modalities used in hand therapy rely on patients' active involvement in rehabilitation and adherence to recommendations. Patient information has also been recognized as an area that should always be addressed by the multidisciplinary team when treating patients with DD.[68] Because patients evaluate their health care providers' intervention, their knowledge and skills, and the interaction between them,[69] tailoring information to the individual patient is important to reach a successful outcome.[70,71] It has been suggested that patients' compliance with the postoperative regime as a whole may influence outcomes[36] and that patients who are more engaged in their health care have better results.[71–73]

SUMMARY

The role of hand therapy in the treatment of DD can differ significantly depending on the patient and the procedure. Thus, hand therapy can be more or less extensive due to factors, such as severity of the disease, type of corrective procedure, phase of tissue healing, phase of the care process, and patients' needs.

Hand therapy as a preventive treatment of DD is uncommon, with limited evidence to support its usefulness. Although the extension deficit can be influenced with an orthotic device, this treatment is demanding for the patient because the orthosis needs to be worn for many hours a day, and the long-term effect on delaying finger contractures is uncertain. Before corrective treatment, a hand therapist can perform an assessment of hand function, activity limitations, and quality of life experienced by an individual to assist in a systematic evaluation of outcomes after treatment. This can also be an opportunity to inform and prepare patients regarding the care process and rehabilitation.

The role of hand therapy is more explicit in connection with corrective treatment where different interventions can be required. The use of orthoses after corrective treatment is not self-evident. In summary, an orthotic intervention is usually part of the hand therapy protocol after corrective procedures for DD, although there is a lack of strong evidence to support this intervention. Nevertheless, it can be argued that previous research does not imply that orthoses are ineffective[27] but perhaps the use of them can be more selective. Additional research is needed, however, to establish indicators for which patients benefit the most from being provided with an orthosis, the optimal orthosis design and the duration of use as well as what other interventions in a hand therapy protocol contribute to maintaining digital joint extension after surgery.

When it comes to evaluation of hand therapy, this involves challenges with multiple treatment modalities (eg, orthoses, exercise, edema control, pain, and/or scar management) that have to be tailored to each patient's problems.[31,38] This individualized approach contrasts starkly with the standardization and control of intervention that is characterized in high-quality research. Hence, the efficacy of hand therapy is difficult to study. Investigation of orthotic interventions for patients with DD has been examined with several RCT studies. For other treatment modalities there is a lack of large, high-quality studies that investigate their efficacy, specifically for patients with DD. Nevertheless, interventions directed toward range of motion, swelling, and pain or scarring are recognized as essential parts of a hand therapy protocol for patients with DD and for recovery of hand function.[31] The intervention provided to patients with DD is thus based on the therapist's clinical reasoning and the patient's needs as well as the available evidence. In the future, further evidence is needed for specific therapy interventions for patients with DD as well as evidence for patients' compliance with those interventions.

REFERENCES

1. Dimick MP, Caro CM, Kasch MC, et al. 2008 practice analysis study of hand therapy. J Hand Ther 2009; 22(4):361–75.
2. IFSHT. IFSHT hand therapy practice profile. Secondary IFSHT hand therapy practice profile. 2010. Available at: https://www.ifsht.org/page/what-hand-therapy. Accessed April 25, 2018.
3. Shih B, Bayat A. Scientific understanding and clinical management of Dupuytren disease. Nat Rev Rheumatol 2010;(6):715–26.
4. Hurst L. Dupuytren's disease: surgical management. In: Skriven T, Osterman A, Fedorczyk J, et al, editors. Rehabilitation of the hand. 6th edition. Philadelphia: Elsevier Mosby; 2011. p. 266–80.
5. Prosser R, Conolly WB. Complications following surgical treatment for Dupuytren's contracture. J Hand Ther 1996;9(4):344–8.
6. Keller JL, Caro CM, Dimick MP, et al. Thirty years of hand therapy: the 2014 practice analysis. J Hand Ther 2016;29(3):222–34.
7. Pratt A, Byrne G. The lived experience of Dupuytren's disease of the hand. J Clin Nurs 2009;18(12): 1793–802.
8. Ball C, Izadi D, Verjee LS, et al. Systematic review of non-surgical treatments for early dupuytren's disease. BMC Musculoskelet Disord 2016;17(1):345.
9. Larocerie-Salgado J, Davidson J. Nonoperative treatment of PIPJ flexion contractures associated with Dupuytren's disease. J Hand Surg Eur Vol 2012;37(8):722–7.
10. Ball C, Nanchahal J. The use of splinting as a non-surgical treatment for Dupuytren's disease: a pilot study. Br Journal of Hand Therapy 2002;(7):76–8.
11. Christie WS, Puhl AA, Lucaciu OC. Cross-frictional therapy and stretching for the treatment of palmar adhesions due to Dupuytren's contracture: a prospective case study. Man Ther 2012;17(5): 479–82.
12. Brauns A, Van Nuffel M, De Smet L, et al. A clinical trial of tension and compression orthoses for Dupuytren contractures. J Hand Ther 2017;30(3): 253–61.
13. Dias JJ, Singh HP, Ullah A, et al. Patterns of recontracture after surgical correction of Dupuytren disease. J Hand Surg 2013;38(10):1987–93.
14. Degreef I, De Smet L. Risk factors in Dupuytren's diathesis: is recurrence after surgery predictable? Acta Orthop Belg 2011;77(1):27–32.
15. Ball C, Pratt A, Nanchahal J. Optimal functional outcome measures for assessing treatment for Dupuytren's disease: a systematic review and recommendations for future practice. BMC Musculoskelet Disord 2013;14(14):131.
16. Rodrigues J, Zhang W, Scammell B, et al. What patients want from the treatment of Dupuytren's disease – is the Unite Rhumatologique des Affections de la Main (URAM) scale relevant? J Hand Surg Eur Vol 2014;39(6):673–5.
17. Beaudreuil J, Lermusiaux J, Teyssedou J, et al. Multi-needle aponeurotomy for advanced Dupuytren's disease: preliminary results of safety and efficacy (MNA 1 study). Joint Bone Spine 2011;78(6): 625–8.
18. Bernabe B, Lasbleiz S, Gerber RA, et al. URAM scale for functional assessment in Dupuytren's disease: a comparative study of its properties. Joint Bone Spine 2014;81(5):441–4.
19. Mohan A, Vadher J, Ismail H, et al. The southampton dupuytren's scoring scheme. J Plast Surg Hand Surg 2014;48(1):28–33.
20. Jerosch-Herold C, Shepstone L, Chojnowski A, et al. Severity of contracture and self-reported disability in patients with Dupuytren's contracture referred for surgery. J Hand Ther 2011;24(1):6–10.

21. Forget NJ, Jerosch-Herold C, Shepstone L, et al. Psychometric evaluation of the Disabilities of the Arm, Shoulder and Hand (DASH) with Dupuytren's contracture: validity evidence using Rasch modeling. BMC Musculoskelet Disord 2014;15:361.

22. Rodrigues J, Zhang W, Scammell B, et al. Validity of the Disabilities of the Arm, Shoulder and Hand patient-reported outcome measure (DASH) and the Quickdash when used in Dupuytren's disease. J Hand Surg Eur Vol 2016;41(6):589–99.

23. Rodrigues JN, Zhang W, Scammell BE, et al. Recovery, responsiveness and interpretability of patient-reported outcome measures after surgery for Dupuytren's disease. J Hand Surg Eur Vol 2017; 42(3):301–9.

24. Engstrand C, Boren L, Liedberg G. Evaluation of activity limitation and digital extension in Dupuytren's contracture three months after fasciectomy and hand therapy interventions. J Hand Ther 2009; 22(1):21–6.

25. Engstrand C, Krevers B, Kvist J. Factors affecting functional recovery after surgery and hand therapy in patients with Dupuytren's disease. J Hand Ther 2015;28(3):255–9.

26. Au-Yong I, Wildin C, Page RE. A review of common practice in Dupuytren Surgery. Tech Hand Up Extrem Surg 2005;9:178–87.

27. Sweet S, Blackmore S. Surgical and therapy update on the management of Dupuytren's disease. J Hand Ther 2014;27(2):77–83.

28. Bainbridge C, Dahlin LB, Szczypa PP, et al. Current trends in the surgical management of Dupuytren's disease in Europe: an analysis of patient charts. Eur Orthop Traumatol 2012;3(1):31–41.

29. Dahlin L, Bainbridge C, Szczypa P, et al. Current trends in the surgical management of Dupuytren's disease in Europe: the surgeon's perspective. Eur Orthop Traumatol 2012;3(1):25–30.

30. Bayat A, McGrouther DA. Management of Dupuytren's disease - clear advice for an elusive condition. Ann R Coll Surg Engl 2006;88:3–8.

31. Engstrand C, Krevers B, Nylander G, et al. Hand function and quality of life before and after fasciectomy for Dupuytren disease. J Hand Surg 2014; 39(7):1333–43.

32. Herweijer H, Dijkstra PU, Nicolai JP, et al. Postoperative hand therapy in Dupuytren's disease. Disabil Rehabil 2007;29(22):1736–41.

33. Fess EE. A history of splinting: to understand the present, view the past. J Hand Ther 2002;15(2):97–132.

34. Larson D, Jerosch-Herold C. Clinical effectiveness of post-operative splinting after surgical release of Dupuytren's contracture: a systematic review. BMC Musculoskelet Disord 2008;9:104.

35. Rodrigues JN, Becker GW, Ball C, et al. Surgery for Dupuytren's contracture of the fingers. Cochrane Database Syst Rev 2015;(12):CD010143.

36. Rives K, Gelberman R, Smith B, et al. Severe contractures of the proximal interphalangeal joint in Dupuytren's disease: results of a prospective trial of operative correction and dynamic extension splinting. J Hand Surg 1992;17A(6):1153–9.

37. Ebskov LB, Boeckstyns ME, Sorensen AI, et al. Results after surgery for severe Dupuytren's contracture: does a dynamic extension splint influence outcome? Scand J Plast Reconstr Surg Hand Surg 2000;34(2):155–60.

38. Jerosch-Herold C, Shepstone L, Chojnowski AJ, et al. Night-time splinting after fasciectomy or dermo-fasciectomy for Dupuytren's contracture: a pragmatic, multi-centre, randomised controlled trial. BMC Musculoskelet Disord 2011;12:136.

39. Collis J, Collocott S, Hing W, et al. The effect of night extension orthoses following surgical release of Dupuytren contracture: a single-center, randomized, controlled trial. J Hand Surg 2013;38(7): 1285–94.

40. Kemler MA, Houpt P, van der Horst CM. A pilot study assessing the effectiveness of postoperative splinting after limited fasciectomy for Dupuytren's disease. J Hand Surg Eur volume 2012;37(8):733–7.

41. Evans RB, Dell PC, Fiolkowski P. A clinical report of the effect of mechanical stress on functional results after fasciectomy for Dupuytren's contracture. J Hand Ther 2002;15(4):331–9.

42. Rivlin M, Osterman M, Jacoby S, et al. The incidence of postoperative flare reaction and tissue complications in Dupuytren's disease using tension-free immobilization. Hand 2014;(9):459–65.

43. Meinel A. Long-term static overnight extension splinting following percutaneous needle fasciotomy. Handchir Mikrochir Plast Chir 2011;43(5):286–8 [in German].

44. Tam L, Chung Y. Needle aponeurotomy for Dupuytren contracture: effectiveness of postoperative night extension splinting. Plast Surg 2016;24(1):23–6.

45. Scherman P, Jenmalm P, Dahlin LB. One-year results of needle fasciotomy and collagenase injection in treatment of Dupuytren's contracture: a two-centre prospective randomized clinical trial. J Hand Surg Eur 2016;41E(6):577–82.

46. Naam N. Functional outcome of collagenase injections compared with fasciectomy in treatment of Dupuytren's contracture. Hand 2013;(8):410–6.

47. Hurst LC, Badalamente MA, Hentz VR, et al. Injectable collagenase clostridium histolyticum for Dupuytren's contracture. N Engl J Med 2009;361(10): 968–79.

48. Degreef I. Collagenase treatment in dupuytren contractures: a review of the current state versus future needs. Rheumatol Ther 2016;3(1):43–51.

49. Mickelson DT, Noland SS, Watt AJ, et al. Prospective randomized controlled trial comparing 1- versus 7-day manipulation following collagenase injection

for dupuytren contracture. J Hand Surg 2014;39(10): 1933–41.

50. Coleman S, Gilpin D, Kaplan FT, et al. Efficacy and safety of concurrent collagenase clostridium histolyticum injections for multiple Dupuytren contractures. J Hand Surg 2014;39(1):57–64.

51. Nydick JA, Olliff BW, Garcia MJ, et al. A comparison of percutaneous needle fasciotomy and collagenase injection for dupuytren disease. J Hand Surg 2013; 38(12):2377–80.

52. Muppavarapu R, Waters M, Leibman M, et al. Clinical outcomes following collagenase injections compared to fasciectomy in the treatment of Dupuytren's contracture. Hand 2015;(10):260–5.

53. Skirven TM, Bachoura A, Jacoby SM, et al. The effect of a therapy protocol for increasing correction of severely contracted proximal interphalangeal joints caused by dupuytren disease and treated with collagenase injection. J Hand Surg 2013; 38(4):684–9.

54. Samargandi OA, Alyouha S, Larouche P, et al. Night orthosis after surgical correction of dupuytren contractures: a systematic review. J Hand Surg 2017; 42(10):839.e1-e10.

55. Huisstede BM, Hoogvliet P, Coert JH, et al. Dupuytren disease: European hand surgeons, hand therapists, and physical medicine and rehabilitation physicians agree on a multidisciplinary treatment guideline: results from the HANDGUIDE study. Plast Reconstr Surg 2013;132(6):964–76.

56. Midgley R. Use of casting motion to mobilize stiffness to regain digital flexion following Dupuytren's fasciectomy. Hand Ther 2010;(15):45–51.

57. Comer GC, Clark SJ, Yao J. Hand therapy modalities for proximal interphalangeal joint stiffness. J Hand Surg 2015;40(11):2293–6.

58. Glassey N. A study of the effect of night extension splintage on post-fasciectomy Dupuytren's patients. Br J Hand Ther 2001;6(3):89–94.

59. Michlovitz S, Harris BA, Watkins MP. Therapy interventions for improving joint range of motion: a systematic review. J Hand Ther 2004;17:118–31.

60. Glasgow C, Tooth LR, Fleming J. Mobilizing the stiff hand: combining theory and evidence to improve clinical outcomes. J Hand Ther 2010;23(4):392–400.

61. Crean S, Gerber R, Hellio Le Graverand M, et al. The efficacy and safety of fasciectomy and fasciotomy for Dupuytren's contracture in European patients: a structured review of published studies. J Hand Surg Eur 2011;36(5):396–407.

62. Badalamente MA, Hurst LC, Benhaim P, et al. Efficacy and safety of collagenase clostridium histolyticum in the treatment of proximal interphalangeal joints in dupuytren contracture: combined analysis of 4 phase 3 clinical trials. J Hand Surg 2015; 40(5):975–83.

63. Evans RB. Therapeutic management of Dupuytren's contracture. In: Skriven T, Osterman A, Fedorczuk J, et al, editors. Rehabilitation of the hand and upper extremity. 6th edition. Philadelphia: Elsevier Mosby; 2011. p. 281–8.

64. Colditz JC. Plaster of Paris: the forgotten hand splinting material. J Hand Ther 2002;15(2):144–57.

65. Denkler K. Surgical complications associated with fasciectomy for dupuytren's disease: a 20-year review of the English literature. Eplasty 2010;10:e15.

66. Villeco JP. Edema: therapist's management. In: Skirven T, Lee Osterman A, Fedorczyk J, et al, editors. Rehabilitation of the hand and upper extremity. 6th edition. Philadelphia: Elsevier Mosby; 2011. p. 845–57.

67. Shin TM, Bordeaux JS. The role of massage in scar management: a literature review. Dermatol Surg 2012;38(3):414–23.

68. Jones L. Scar management in hand therapy - is our practice evidence based? Br J Hand Ther 2005; 10(2):40–6.

69. Pomey MP, Ghadiri DP, Karazivan P, et al. Patients as partners: a qualitative study of patients' engagement in their health care. PLoS One 2015;10(4): e0122499.

70. Moorhead J, Cooper C, Moorhead P. Personality type and patient education in hand therapy. J Hand Ther 2011;24(2):147–53.

71. Engstrand C, Kvist J, Krevers B. Patients' perspective on surgical intervention for Dupuytren's disease - experiences, expectations and appraisal of results. Disabil Rehabil 2016;36(26):1–12.

72. Gruber JS, Hageman M, Neuhaus V, et al. Patient activation and disability in upper extremity illness. J Hand Surg 2014;39(7):1378–83.

73. Hibbard JH, Greene J. What the evidence shows about patient activation: better health outcomes and care experiences; fewer data on costs. Health Aff 2013;32(2):207–14.

Treatment of Recurrent Dupuytren Disease

Frederick Thomas D. Kaplan, MD*, Nicholas E. Crosby, MD

KEYWORDS

- Dupuytren disease • Recurrence • Outcomes • Collagenase *Clostridium histolyticum*
- Aponeurotomy • Dermofasciectomy • Continuous passive elongation

KEY POINTS

- A consistent definition of recurrent Dupuytren contracture is necessary. We support "a passive extension deficit of more than 20° for at least one of the treated joints, in the presence of a palpable cord, compared with the result obtained at time 0."
- Determination of best treatment option is based on volar soft tissue condition, neurovascular function, contracture severity, and patient expectations/willingness to participate in postoperative management.
- Patients with well-defined cords are best candidates for collagenase and percutaneous aponeurotomy.
- Severe contractures with significant scarring and diffuse fibromatosis are best suited for dermofasciectomy and continuous passive elongation.

 Video content accompanies this article at http://www.hand.theclinics.com.

INTRODUCTION

One of the more difficult parts in caring for patients with Dupuytren contracture is the incurable and unpredictable nature of the disease. Outcomes of treatment are highly variable in the short and long term because of differences in patient biology and treatment methods. Managing recurrent disease is even more challenging, requiring surgeons to have many tools at their disposal. This article highlights options for the treatment of disease recurrence following initial management with needle aponeurotomy, clostridial collagenase, or surgical fasciectomy.

DIAGNOSIS OF RECURRENT DUPUYTREN DISEASE

Determining the best treatment of a patient with recurrent Dupuytren disease begins with a thorough assessment of the patient's current situation, prior treatments, and expectations. It is also important to determine the time course of recurrence, and whether the contracture is a true recurrence caused by redevelopment of contracted fibromatosis in the previously treated area or caused by residual secondary changes involving the joint, periarticular structures, and tendon function.

The definition of recurrence itself varies significantly in the literature. Werker and colleagues[1] highlighted this problem in 2011, reviewing 218 studies on the treatment of Dupuytren disease, finding only 21 studies with definitions of recurrence, quantitative results for contracture correction and recurrence, and a sample size of at least 20 patients. There was a wide variety in the definition of recurrence, and in all but one of the studies, definitions of recurrence were qualitative, highlighting the need for a consensus definition. In a prospective trial assessing the safety and efficacy of clostridial collagenase, Hurst and colleagues[2] defined recurrence as "an increase in joint

Disclosure Statement: Speakers Bureau for Endo Pharmaceuticals (F.T.D. Kaplan). None (N.E. Crosby).
Indiana Hand to Shoulder Center, 8501 Harcourt Road, Indianapolis, IN 46260, USA
* Corresponding author.
E-mail address: tkaplan@ihtsc.com

Hand Clin 34 (2018) 403–415
https://doi.org/10.1016/j.hcl.2018.03.009

contracture to 20° or more in the presence of a palpable cord." This same definition was also reached by Felici and colleagues,[3] who in 2014 surveyed 24 hand surgeons from 17 countries who confirmed the need for a clear definition of recurrence that could be applied to any length of follow-up. They concluded "a passive extension deficit of more than 20° for at least one of the treated joints, in the presence of a palpable cord, compared to the result obtained at time 0 represented the definition of recurrence."

When taking a patient's history, it is important to get as much detail as possible regarding what treatment they had on the finger, whether it was fully straight initially, how long it took for the contracture to redevelop, and any complications they had. These details can provide information useful in deciding what future treatment options may be best. It is also useful to know if they had any other fingers treated and how those behaved.

Examination of the hand should include the location of prior incisions, range of motion, neurovascular status, and presence of palpable cords and nodules. Joint contracture is measured as the passive extension deficit (PED) at the metacarpophalangeal (MCP), proximal interphalangeal (PIP), and distal interphalangeal (DIP) joints. Be aware of dynamism, where the position of one joint can alter the PED of the adjacent joint.[4] This typically occurs when a pretendinous cord crosses both the MCP and PIP joints, particularly in the small and ring fingers where there is increased motion at the carpometacarpal joints.

The quality of the skin and consistency of the fibromatosis have significant impact on the treatment options best suited to the patient. Patients may present with clear recurrent disease: a well-developed cord and corresponding contracture. Less invasive treatment options, such as percutaneous fasciotomy and clostridial collagenase injections, are best suited in these patients, although all options remain viable. At the other end of the spectrum, patients may have a recurrent contracture with diffuse scarring and fibrosis, but without a clearly identifiable cord. In these situations, more aggressive treatments are often required, such as dermofasciectomy or staged fasciectomy following prolonged soft-tissue distraction.

Finally, secondary adaptive changes often occur, particularly with severe PIP joint involvement. In addition to capsular contracture, patients may develop boutonnière deformity because of extensor tendon attenuation, volar subluxation of the lateral bands, and oblique retinacular ligament tightness. In these patients it is common to find abnormal thickened fascia along the lateral digital sheets, extending past the typical cord insertion on the middle phalanx, connecting into the extensor apparatus.

TREATMENT OPTIONS

Patients with recurrent Dupuytren contracture are treated by any of the treatments discussed in this issue. Decision on which treatment is most appropriate is best determined through shared decision making with the patient. Surgeons should understand what factors the patient believes are most important and fully discuss the options with respect to their efficacy, recurrence rates, complications, and postoperative management. Certainly, in each case there is unpredictability in outcomes, and patients should be guided away from options whose risks outweigh the benefits (eg, collagenase injection in a patient with a 90° recurrent PIP contracture with diffuse fibrosis and no clearly identifiable cord).

Treatment with percutaneous techniques, including needle aponeurotomy and collagenase injection, is best suited to those patients with recurrent disease that is well defined. Additionally, in patients with severe PIP contractures, it is likely there are significant secondary factors contributing to the contracture. Release of the offending cord or cords will likely lead to only partial correction, and maximal improvement will require a diligent rehabilitation program.

Patients with recurrent disease and severe contracture, particularly in the setting of significant scar tissue and diffuse, thick fibromatosis, are best managed with more robust interventions to maximize reduction in contracture and minimize recurrence. In addition to standard fasciectomy, adjuvant procedures, such as skin grafting (dermofasciectomy), flap coverage, and initial continuous passive elongation, are more often used in these situations.

Salvage procedures mostly play a role for patients with multiple recurrences, severe PIP contractures, neurovascular compromise, and severe scarring. In these instances, PIP fusion or amputation may be the best option for the patient.

TREATMENT OF RECURRENCE WITH NEEDLE APONEUROTOMY

As in primary disease, percutaneous needle aponeurotomy for recurrent Dupuytren should be considered for the appropriate patient (See Kate E. Elzinga and Michael J. Morharts' article, "Needle Aponeurotomy for Dupuytren Disease", in this issue). Little research has been reported on the treatment of recurrent Dupuytren disease with needle aponeurotomy. van Rijssen and Werker[5] reported their experience in treating recurrent disease in 40 patients with needle apo-neurotomy after previous needle aponeurotomy or open fasciectomy. They showed promising re-sults in contracture reduction of 76% (MCP joint greater than PIP joint), 46% recurrence at 4.4 years, and no complications including neuro-vascular injury. In a follow-up study, the senior author reported on needle aponeurotomy treat-ment of third, fourth, and fifth recurrence treat-ments in 16 fingers.[6] Contracture correction rates and recurrence after third and fourth treatments were similar to those after primary and secondary treatment, but a fifth treatment of needle aponeur-otomy showed poor results with only 27% reduc-tion in PED, compared with 73% reduction for third, and 63% for fourth treatments.

Indications for needle aponeurotomy include recurrent disease with greater MCP involvement than PIP involvement, with well-defined cords that are readily palpated. The surgeon should avoid treatment in areas with significant scar tis-sue that obscures cord features, and in patients with prior neurovascular compromise that limits the ability to adequately assess fine touch sensa-tion during the procedure.

Surgical Technique

- The surgical technique for percutaneous nee-dle aponeurotomy can vary among practi-tioners, but basic principles are often uniform. The procedure may be done in a semi-sterile or full sterile setting, either in the clinic or an operative suite. The patient should be respon-sive with an ability to express pain or neuro-logic changes. Local anesthetic in only the dermal/epidermal skin layers should be used to maintain sensation in the digital nerves.
- Once the hand is prepared, use a 30-gauge needle to injection local anesthetic into the dermal and epidermal skin layers. The fingertip is assessed for light touch sensation initially and throughout the entire case. Trac-tion should be placed on the cord by pulling on it via skin or nodules distal to the treatment point. A 25-gauge needle is then passed through the skin and obliquely under the skin to open a space between the skin and the cord. The needle is then swept side-to-side through the cord from superficial to deep until a palpable release is noted.
- If neurologic changes are noted during the needle sweep, the fingertip should be as-sessed for sensation. If sensation is present, caution should be used but the procedure may continue. If sensation is absent, the pro-cedure should be abandoned in favor of an open procedure or repeat needle fasciectomy at a later date.
- The tendon is evaluated during the procedure by asking the patient to lightly flex and extend the digit. If the needle is too deep and into the tendon, the needle moves with finger motion. Otherwise, the procedure may continue.
- Releases should proceed from distal to prox-imal. Great care should be taken when pre-forming the procedure distal to the MCP joint because spiral cords may alter the anatomy significantly. As noted by Popovic and col-leagues[7] the neurovascular bundle position may be even more dramatically centralized by a spiral cord or scar tissue after a prior treat-ment. This can also occur more proximally than typical and great care should be taken during this and other percutaneous techniques.
- Avoid needle access points in nodules (diffi-cult release) and skin creases (excessive skin tearing).
- Use fresh needles as often as appropriate to maintain sharp dissection and adequate tactile feedback.
- Repeatedly assess distal sensation during the procedure.
- Final manipulation is done stepwise from PIP to MCP with compensatory proximal joint flexion to reduce stress on skin.
- A soft dressing is applied. No specific therapy or splinting regimen is required.

Postoperative Care

- Dressing is removed the following day.
- Patients are instructed to begin home range-of-motion exercises and gentle passive stretching.
- Night splinting may be beneficial in some situ-ations, particularly for severe PIP contrac-tures, although evidence for the efficacy of splinting is lacking.
- Warn patient against heavy grip or use for at least 1 to 2 weeks after the procedure.

Complications

- Neurovascular injury is possible but should be limited by close monitoring of sensation dur-ing the procedure. Rates of neurapraxia of 2% to 3% and nerve division of 0.4% have been reported.[8]
- Skin tears are the most common complica-tion, particularly at palm creases.
  - Skin tears are treated by daily cleaning with warm soapy water and dressing with a petroleum-based antibiotic ointment on the open wound until healed.

- Tendon rupture either intraoperatively or during heavy use postoperatively (higher risk with lower gauge needles).

TREATMENT OF RECURRENCE WITH COLLAGENASE

Patients with recurrent contracture, regardless of whether the initial treatment was with collagenase, needle aponeurotomy, or fasciectomy, may be candidates for collagenase. The only contraindication is in patients with a history of hypersensitivity to previous collagenase use. Collagenase works best in situations where there is limited scarring, such as digits with prior percutaneous treatment, and those postfasciectomy with clearly defined cords. Bear and colleagues[9] reported the results of 51 patients retreated with collagenase after recurrence of contracture. A total of 57% of joints achieved contracture of 5° or less (65% of MCP and 45% of PIP joints), with average pretreatment MCP contracture of 40° and PIP contracture of 46°.

The technique for administration of collagenase in recurrent cases is like that for primary disease (See Marie A. Badalamente and Lawrence C. Hursts' article, "Development of Collagenase Treatment for Dupuytren Disease," in this issue). The crucial first step is to determine which cords are responsible for which joint contractures. For example, a pretendinous cord can become a central cord resulting in both MCP and PIP contracture. Another common scenario is a lateral digital or abductor digiti minimi cord causing a PIP and DIP contracture. Because each collagenase treatment is for a particular joint, the cord configuration often determines whether all contractures in a finger can be treated with one injection, or if multiple injections are required.

Preferred Technique

- Injection
  - Inject planned sites of injection with local anesthesia superficial to the cord. By reducing the pain of the collagenase injection, it is easier to keep the patient's hand still, and ensure an intralesional injection of the cord.
  - Avoid injecting near skin creases. This can lead to a higher skin tear rate.
  - For thicker and/or longer cords, consider injecting the full amount of collagenase provided in the vial (0.9 mg). This amount is off-label. Reconstitute for MCP or PIP depending on planned sites of injection but spread the injection over four or five locations along the length of the cord.
  - Be careful when injecting abductor digiti minimi and lateral digital cords distal to the proximal digital flexion crease. The risk of collateral tendon damage is higher as the separation between the cord and tendon sheath narrows. Keep the injection intralesional, and if resistance during injection is lost, stop injecting and move to a new area in the cord.
  - For patients with prior skin grafting, avoid injection under the graft. Graft loss has been described following collagenase injection,[10] although careful technique may prevent this complication.[11]
- Manipulation
  - Use local anesthesia to ensure patient is comfortable.
  - Use a stepwise approach (Video 1).
    - Extend PIP joint with MCP flexed.
    - Extend MCP joint with PIP flexed.
    - Perform combined extension of both joints.
    - With tension on the finger, palpate and apply pressure along the cord in areas of injection to further break down longitudinal bands.
  - Watch for darkening areas of skin heralding impending skin tear and cover with gauze (**Fig. 1**).
  - If cord rupture does not occur, and/or there continues to be significant contracture with a palpable cord, a second injection can be planned, given with a minimum of 4 weeks between injections.

Postinjection Care

- Patients are instructed to begin edema control and active range-of-motion exercises immediately. Use of a compression glove for the first several weeks is helpful.

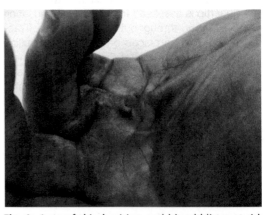

Fig. 1. Area of skin bruising and blood blister at risk for developing into skin tear during manipulation.

- A hand-based extension splint is worn nightly for 4 weeks. In cases of severe PIP contracture, splinting may be continued for 3 to 4 months or until tissue homeostasis occurs.
- Patients are advised to avoid forceful grasping for 3 to 4 weeks, to lessen the risk of flexor tendon rupture, particularly when the small finger PIP has been treated.
- The finger is re-evaluated at 1 to 2 weeks postinjection.
  - If patient continues to have a significant contracture with a palpable cord, or a secondary joint to treat, the next injection is planned, waiting the requisite 4 weeks between injections.
  - If there continues to be PIP joint contracture, without a palpable cord that could benefit from further injection, an aggressive PIP rehabilitation protocol is begun.
    - Skirven and colleagues[12] compared their results of patients with PIP contractures greater than 40° treated with one injection with published results of similar contractures treated in the Collagenase Option for Reduction of Dupuytren (CORD) I and II studies. In the 22 patients studied using their rehabilitation protocol, they found a higher percentage gained a reduction in contracture to less than 5° (55% compared with 22% for CORD 1 and 25% for CORD 2); and mean contracture improved from 56° at baseline to 7° at 4 weeks (compared with 54° to 28° in CORD I and 56° to 33° in CORD II).

Complications

- Edema, ecchymosis, and pain occur frequently following collagenase injection.
- Pruritis and lymphadenopathy occur in 10% to 20% of cases, with higher rates of pruritis in patients with prior collagenase treatment.[9,13]
- Skin tear
  - Skin tears have been reported in 13% of patients treated with collagenase for recurrent contracture.[9]
  - Patients with skin tears are instructed to wash the hand with soapy water daily, and to keep the wound moist with a petroleum-based antibiotic ointment, avoiding the surrounding skin.
  - Most skin tears heal uneventfully within 2 to 3 weeks via secondary intention (**Fig. 2**).
- Flexor tendon rupture
  - Flexor tendon rupture is a rare complication, with reported incidence of 0.05%.[14]
  - There is no known added risk when treating patients with recurrent contracture. However, in these cases, it is critical to remember the importance of only injecting into well-defined cords, and keeping the injection intralesional.

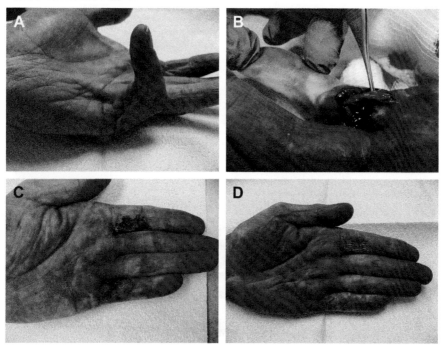

Fig. 2. Skin tear occurring during manipulation 2 days after injection for MCP contracture of 60° and PIP contracture of 60°. (*A*) Pretreatment contracture. (*B*) Tear with ruptured cord. (*C*) Tear 14 days later. (*D*) Tear at 4 weeks.

Illustrative Case

A 49-year-old man was initially treated for right ring finger MCP contracture of 30° with collagenase in 2010 (**Fig. 3**A). The patient had complete correction of contracture following manipulation (**Fig. 3**B). In 2017, the patient reported recurrent contracture over the past several years. On examination the patient had a well-defined pretendinous cord with MCP contracture of 40° and PIP contracture of 40° (**Fig. 3**C). He requested retreatment with collagenase and had successful rupture of the cord with restoration of full extension at the MCP joint and mild PIP contracture of 10° (**Fig. 3**D, E).

TREATMENT OF RECURRENCE WITH FASCIECTOMY

Open palmar fasciectomy is a mainstay of treatment of recurrent Dupuytren disease. Several factors associated with recurrence may support open surgery in place of percutaneous options, including significant scar formation, altered anatomy, and poorly defined disease tissue. In cases of severe joint contracture where soft tissue release of periarticular structures is likely to be required, open fasciectomy is indicated. One must also consider poor skin condition and scar formation as an indication for open fasciectomy. In these circumstances, Z-plasties, skin grafts, flaps, and other options must be considered. Finally, recurrent disease often exhibits flattened and poorly defined fibrotic tissue that is best treated with direct visualization and removal of the pathology. Open fasciectomy continues to serve as the gold standard for the treatment of primary and recurrent Dupuytren disease and should be considered in all cases of recurrence.

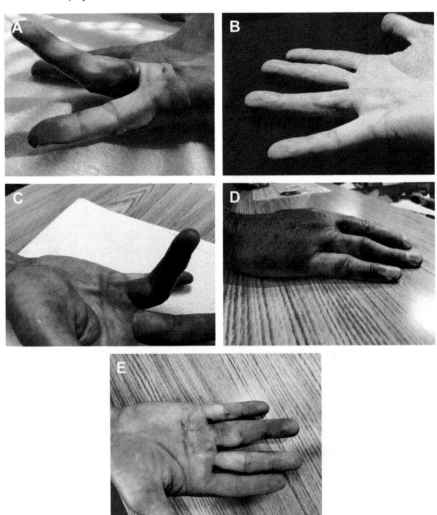

Fig. 3. Treatment of recurrent contracture with collagenase. (*A*) Initial contracture of 30°. (*B*) Full correction at 5 weeks. (*C*) Recurrent contracture before retreatment with collagenase 7 years later. (*D, E*) Correction obtained following manipulation.

Outcomes after open fasciectomy are overall positive as noted in multiple historical and recent publications. Reliable and satisfactory results are expected after fasciectomy for recurrent disease. In a study of 16 patients undergoing fasciectomy three or more times on a single hand, Konneker and colleagues[15] found an average increased PIP range of motion of 59°, although 43% had delayed wound healing, and 25% sustained arterial injury requiring reconstruction. In 18 patients with 22 fingers operated on for recurrence, Spies and colleagues[16] found, with mean follow-up of 94 months, that most patients obtain grip and pinch strength of at least 90% compared with the contralateral side, and DASH (Disabilities of the Arm, Shoulder, and Hand) scores of less than 15.

Preoperative Planning

- A careful history of prior treatments should be obtained.
- Evaluation of previous skin incisions.
- Areas of potential skin complications should be noted and skin grafting, flaps, or dermofasciectomy considered.

Preferred Technique

- The palm should be opened proximal to the palpable disease.
- Dissection is initially carried out from proximal to distal.
- Neurovascular structures are identified and followed starting in the midpalm region. Scar formation in the palm after prior surgery can make structure identification and elevation of skin flaps difficult.
- More common in revision surgery than primary, spiral cords and natatory cords often obscure the anatomy near the proximal flexion creases of the digits. If the neurovascular structures become unidentifiable, distal to proximal dissection should be initiated around the PIP or DIP joint level and followed back to meet the proximal dissection.
- Z-plasty should be planned as necessary for any longitudinal scar lengthening.
- MCP or PIP joint releases can also be considered and completed once the fasciectomy is complete.
- Incisions may be left open to heal via secondary intention. We typically make a transverse incision along the distal palmar crease, continuing in Bruner fashion into the digits. Even in severe contractures, the Bruner incision can almost always be closed; however, we commonly leave part of the transverse palmar incision open.

Postoperative Care

- No consistent consensus exists regarding rehabilitation and splinting after open fasciectomy.
- Splinting is often used at least short term to maintain extension between range-of-motion exercises and provide comfort for the patient.
- We typically splint in extension (or progressive extension based on intraoperative correction and concern for neurovascular structure tightness) full-time for 4 to 6 weeks, then nighttime only for several months.

Complications

- Nerve laceration is reported in 2% to 5% of surgeries, with increased rates when treating PIP contractures greater than 60°.[17] Roush and Stern[18] reported 68% of fingers treated for recurrent disease had a tactile deficit at final follow-up, and 11% of fingers had no sensibility.
- Digital arterial injury is also more common in recurrent surgery than primary fasciectomy (11%–30% vs 1%–3%).[19,20]
- Flare reaction can lead to significant postoperative swelling, pain, and recurrent contracture, and this occurs in 5% of cases.[20]
- Infection is reported in 5% to 10% of patients.[17,20]
- Skin slough and necrosis occurs in 8% of primary surgeries and 12% of revisions.[20]
- Aggressive resection of pulleys during flexor sheath release can often lead to bowstringing and permanent motion limitations.

Illustrative Case

A 63-year-old man presented with recurrence of contracture of the left index finger 2 years after treatment with collagenase. He had been initially treated for an MCP contracture of 25° and a PIP contracture of 35° with two injections. After injection he improved to 0° at the MCP joint and 15° at the PIP joint (**Fig. 4**A, B); however, he had recurrent contracture associated with a thick nodule over the proximal phalanx. Two years following collagenase, his MCP contracture was 35° and PIP contracture 25° (**Fig. 4**C). Considering the thick, nodular disease, it was believed that fasciectomy would lead to the best correction of contracture and least risk of recurrence. At surgery, the area of nodularity was clearly identified and represented the area of recurrent fibromatosis in the area of previous injection (**Fig. 4**D). The tissue planes were easily dissected, and the patient healed uneventfully (**Fig. 4**E, F).

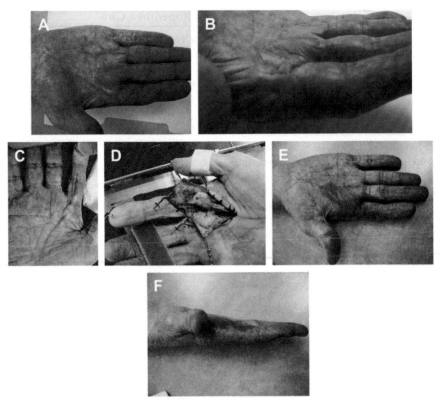

Fig. 4. Treatment of recurrence following collagenase with fasciectomy. (*A, B*) Mild residual contracture of PIP joint following collagenase injection. (*C*) Recurrent nodular fibromatosis with contracture of MCP and PIP joints. (*D*) Area of thick, unorganized fibromatosis in area of previous injection. (*E, F*) One month after fasciectomy with maintenance of correction.

TREATMENT OF RECURRENCE WITH DERMOFASCIECTOMY

Dermofasciectomy was first suggested by Piulachs in 1952 as a means to reduce recurrence after surgical excision.[21] Hueston[22] popularized the technique and suggested it should be considered in four situations: (1) longitudinal skin deficiency following correction of flexion deformity, (2) for recurrent contractures when the skin is densely involved, (3) when the skin is devitalized during surgery, and (4) as a primary procedure in young patients with strong Dupuytren diathesis.

Outcomes of dermofasciectomy have overall been positive when compared with standard fasciectomy. Brotherston and colleagues[23] reported on 34 patients with 5- to 8-year follow-up and saw no recurrences. In a series of 103 patients with 143 rays treated for diffuse disease with skin involvement, Armstrong and colleagues[24] found recurrence in 12 rays with mean follow-up of 5.8 years. Chen and colleagues[25] treated 40 hands with dermofasciectomy and 28 hands with fasciectomy alone, finding no recurrence in the dermofasciectomy group, but 13 recurrences in the fasciectomy group.

In patients treated with dermofasciectomy for recurrent disease, Villani and colleagues[26] found at an average follow-up of 8.8 years only 3 of 23 patients had recurrence. However, not all results have been uniformly positive. In a prospective, randomized study comparing "firebreak" skin graft with Z-plasty closure in 90 fingers, Ullah and colleagues[27] found no significant difference in recurrent contracture of the PIP joint over the 3-year period of follow-up, with 13.6% in the dermofasciectomy group and 11% in the Z-plasty group, although what defined a recurrence was not stated.

Our practice is to consider dermofasciectomy in patients with recurrent contracture with diffuse, poorly localized fibromatosis, particularly in the setting of PIP joint contracture greater than 75°. In these situations, we often perform dermofasciectomy in a staged fashion, after initial reversal of contracture with a continuous passive elongation device (Digit Widget).

Preferred Technique

- Surgery is performed under regional anesthesia with a brachial plexus block.

- Skin is excised over the digit from the proximal digital flexion crease to the PIP or DIP joint flexion crease, and from midlateral line to midlateral line (**Fig. 5**F).
- Incision is carried proximally as needed to expose the entire area of disease recurrence and abnormal fascia.
- After careful identification of both neurovascular bundles, all diseased fascia is excised. In the small finger, the abductor digiti minimi cord is always identified and excised, including distal extensions into the extensor mechanism, lateral digital sheet, and retrovascular cords.
- If residual PIP contracture is present, sequential release is performed, with care taken to avoid overzealous dissection, which can lead to PIP hyperextension.
  - Tip: first open the flexor sheath transversely between the A2 and A3 pulleys, then slowly manipulate the PIP joint into extension. If necessary, a second transverse opening is made distal to the A3 pulley.
  - If neutral extension is achieved, but there is significant rebound, identify and release contracted fascia lateral to the PIP joint. Often diseased tissue connects to the extensor mechanism.
  - If significant contracture remains, sequentially release the checkrein ligaments, distal

to the arterial ladder branches, then repeat the gentle passive manipulation. Rarely, the accessory collateral ligaments and subsequent partial release of the proper collateral ligaments may be necessary.
  - Consider pinning the PIP joint in extension for 2 to 3 weeks.
- Harvest a full-thickness skin graft from the groin or medial elbow, avoiding hair-bearing skin. Suture graft in place with a tie-over bolster. The graft can be pie-crusted to help prevent hematoma, which can contribute to graft loss.

Postoperative Care

- Patients are seen 7 to 10 days after surgery for suture removal and initiation of motion exercises with interval extension splinting.
- Once the wounds are fully healed, scar remodeling and passive flexion is begun, with addition of dynamic flexion splints as needed.

Complications

- Patients undergoing revision fasciectomy have a higher intraoperative complication rate, with an approximately 10-fold higher rate of digital nerve and artery injury (1.7% vs 25.7% for nerve; 3.1% vs 17% for artery).[20]

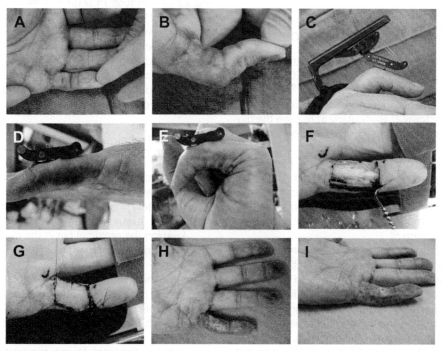

Fig. 5. Treatment of recurrent contracture with continuous passive elongation followed by dermofasciectomy. (*A*, *B*) Recurrent contracture before treatment. (*C*) Day of Digit Widget application. (*D*, *E*) Active motion 8 weeks later at time of device removal. (*F*, *G*) Dermofasciectomy. (*H*, *I*) Five weeks after surgery. (*Courtesy of* [*C*] Hand Biomechanics Lab, Sacramento, CA.)

- Dermofasciectomy has similar complication rates to fasciectomy, other than risk of graft loss and skin contracture.[17,21,27]

Illustrative Case

A 59-year-old right-handed man previously treated with left ring and small finger fasciectomy 3 years ago, and revision fasciectomy with skin grafting 2 years ago, presented with recurrent left small finger PIP contracture of 50° with diffuse scar/fibromatosis (**Fig. 5**A, B). Because of the secondary recurrence, severe contracture, and poorly localized disease, we suggested a two-stage treatment protocol. Patient was first treated with a continuous passive elongation device (Digit Widget) for 8 weeks (**Fig. 5**C). Patient's contracture decreased to 10° in the first 2 weeks, and to 5° by 6 weeks. During this period, he was instructed to perform oblique retinacular ligament stretches and interval PIP joint flexion exercises. At 8 weeks, the fixator was removed and a dermofasciectomy performed (**Fig. 5**D–G). At the time of surgery, after removal of the diseased tissue, full extension of the digit was achieved. Patient began therapy with interval extension splinting, edema control, and flexion exercises. At 5 weeks postoperatively, patient had a mild residual flexion contracture and excellent active motion of the finger (**Fig. 5**H, I, Video 2).

TREATMENT OF RECURRENCE WITH CONTINUOUS PASSIVE ELONGATION

Treatment of severe recurrent Dupuytren disease, particularly in patients with a total PED of greater than 90° (Tubiana stage III or IV),[28] has been shown to have a higher complication rate with revision fasciectomy.[17] Particularly at risk are the digital nerves and arteries.[19,20] Safely dissecting the digital nerve and artery out of the recurrent fascia and scar is extremely difficult, and made even more arduous in cases where the joints are severely contracted. Damage can lead to permanent numbness and even digital ischemia that may necessitate amputation or emergent revascularization.[29]

Preliminary elongation of the contracted joint and periarticular structures was first suggested by Messina[30] in 1989 as a means to reduce the risk of amputation. In addition to the fascia, there are multiple other contracted structures in these fingers, including the collateral ligaments, check-reins and volar plate, flexor theca, and skin. Through continuous distraction, Bailey and colleagues[31] found that there is increased collagen degradation and new collagen synthesis, suggesting actual remodeling of the shortened tissues.

Unfortunately, following removal of the extension device, recontracture typically occurs as the disease process resumes, therefore subsequent fasciectomy is necessary.[32]

Results of fasciectomy after continuous passive elongation have been positive. In a series of 119 fingers in 86 patients, Messina and Messina[33] reported good or excellent functional results in 85% of cases with mean follow-up of 4 years. Craft and colleagues[34] compared fasciectomy with ligament release (20 digits with mean contracture of 55.9°) versus preliminary distraction with the Digit Widget followed by fasciectomy (17 digits with mean contracture of 67.6°). With average follow-up of 18 months, they found significantly improved correction in the distraction group of 53.4°, compared with 31.4° in the fasciectomy with ligament release group. White and colleagues[35] reported their results of initial passive elongation using an external fixator followed by fasciectomy in 38 digits. The second stage, performed 4 weeks after placement of the external fixator, was a dermofasciectomy in all patients. With an average follow-up of 20.6 months, the average PIP contracture improved from 75° to 37°. Most frequent complication was pin track infection, occurring in eight digits.

We consider preliminary passive continuous elongation in patients with recurrent severe contractures with total PED greater than 135° and/or PIP contracture greater than 75°. In patients with limited dermal involvement, we follow with a standard fasciectomy, whereas in patients with diffuse disease and skin involvement we perform a dermofasciectomy. Contraindications to the procedure are underlying joint arthritis or patients with risk of poor compliance with the elongation device.

Preferred Technique (Digit Widget)

- Performed in a surgical suite under digital block anesthesia with fluoroscopic guidance.
- Provided drill guide is placed on the dorsum of the middle phalanx, along the dorsal midlongitudinal axis, and the predrill pins placed, keeping the proximal pin in the metaphysis.
- The pins are sequentially removed and replaced with threaded pins, being careful to stop each pin flush with the volar cortex to avoid irritation or damage to the flexor tendons.
- The pin block is attached to the pins, maintaining at least 5 mm of space between the skin and the block to accommodate swelling.
- Three different strength elastic bands are included (light, medium, heavy). We typically begin with a single medium band.

Postoperative Care

- Patients are instructed to change the elastic band, and clean pin sites daily.
- Overaggressive stretching can lead to significant finger swelling and pain. Patients are begun with a medium band. If this is causing significant pain, patients are instructed to switch to a light band. Conversely, if limited improvement is being seen, or gains are plateauing, patients move to a heavy band, or double bands.
- Patients should perform active flexion exercises throughout the day and may remove the elastic band temporarily if needed.
- If MCP joint hyperextension is present, this must be prevented during treatment with use of the antihyperextension strap.
- Many patients see significant improvement within 2 weeks; however, the device should continue to be used for a least 2 weeks after maximum PIP extension is achieved. Typical duration of use is 4 to 8 weeks.
- Removal of the device can be done preoperatively, at the time of revision fasciectomy, or kept in place to help maintain extension postfasciectomy. Comparison of these options has not been done, so optimal timing is not known.

Complications

- Pin tract infection is the most frequent complication occurring in 2 of 17 cases by Craft and colleagues.[34]
- Overaggressive stretching can lead to soft tissue swelling and skin irritation from impingement on the device.
- Inaccurate pin placement can lead to iatrogenic fracture or flexor tendon irritation.

Illustrative Case

Our patient developed recurrent contracture of the left small finger MCP joint of 10° and PIP joint of 60° 4 years after initial subtotal fasciectomy (**Fig. 6**A, B). Evaluation of the finger revealed significant nodular disease and diffuse fibromatosis believed best addressed by a two-stage procedure. A continuous passive elongation device was placed before planned revision fasciectomy (**Fig. 6**C). Eight days after device application the patient's PIP contracture was reduced to 5°. Four weeks after placement, device removal and revision fasciectomy were performed, with excision of the pretendonous cord (**Fig. 6**D–F). Six weeks following fasciectomy, the patient had maintained full extension (**Fig. 6**G–H).

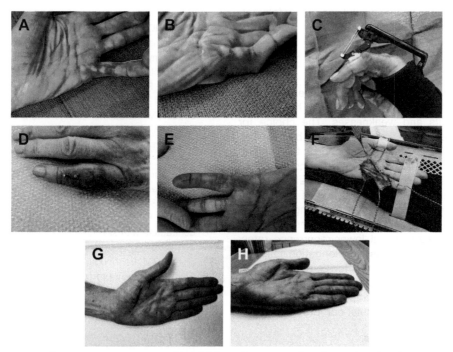

Fig. 6. Treatment of recurrent contracture with initial continuous passive elongation. (*A, B*) Recurrent contracture before treatment. (*C*) Placement of device. (*D, E*) Four weeks after device placement full extension is restored. (*F*) Revision fasciectomy with pretendinous cord dissected and released proximally. (*G, H*) Full extension maintained 6 weeks following fasciectomy. (*Courtesy of* [*C*] Hand Biomechanics Lab, Sacramento, CA.)

SALVAGE PROCEDURES

In certain situations, attempts to improve motion in a finger afflicted by recurrent Dupuytren disease and contracture may be unlikely to provide better function. Digits that have previously underwent multiple surgeries may be best treated with a joint fusion or amputation. These salvage procedures are indicated for patients who have already failed revision surgery and have significant scar contracture, PIP joint arthrofibrosis or arthritis, loss of sensibility, or vascular insufficiency.

PIP arthrodesis is best reserved for those patients with severe PIP contractures with diffuse volar scarring and preserved sensibility. The joint is approached dorsally, and sufficient bone is removed to allow for fusion at the desired angle (typically 40° for ring finger and 45° for small finger). By avoiding volar dissection, and using bony shortening to increase extension, neurovascular injury is prevented. In cases where recurrent cords are present, a limited fasciectomy may be necessary, in addition to PIP fusion, to prevent progressive MCP and/or DIP joint contracture.

Digital amputation is most often performed for patients with severe recurrent contractures who have failed multiple previous treatments. These patients have fingers that may be impairing hygiene, provide no functional benefit, and whose prognosis for improvement is poor. Often the finger may be numb, painful, or cold-intolerant. Amputation for these patients often leads to a more functional hand.

SUMMARY

Treatment of recurrent Dupuytren disease is challenging. Multiple options exist, each having relative benefits and weaknesses. The choice for optimal treatment is made on a case-by-case basis, with shared decision making by the patient. Percutaneous and enzymatic techniques are best reserved for patients with well-defined recurrent disease and offer the benefit of quicker recovery with minimal or no scarring. Surgical treatments have higher risks of neurovascular injury and scarring, but lower recurrence rates. Staged continuous passive elongation followed by dermofasciectomy may lower neurovascular injury and improve outcomes. Salvage procedures may be necessary in patients with poor tissue beds and neurovascular compromise.

SUPPLEMENTARY DATA

Supplementary data related to this article can be found online at https://doi.org/10.1016/j.hcl.2018.03.009.

REFERENCES

1. Werker PM, Pess GM, van Rijssen AL, et al. Correction of contracture and recurrence rates of Dupuytren contracture following invasive treatment: the importance of clear definitions. J Hand Surg Am 2012;37(10):2095–105.e7.
2. Hurst LC, Badalamente MA, Hentz VR, et al. Injectable collagenase Clostridium histolyticum for Dupuytren's contracture. N Engl J Med 2009;361(10):968–79.
3. Felici N, Marcoccio I, Giunta R, et al. Dupuytren contracture recurrence project: reaching consensus on a definition of recurrence. Handchir Mikrochir Plast Chir 2014;46(6):350–4.
4. Rodrigues JN, Zhang W, Scammell BE, et al. Dynamism in Dupuytren's contractures. J Hand Surg Eur Vol 2015;40(2):166–70.
5. van Rijssen AL, Werker PM. Percutaneous needle fasciotomy for recurrent Dupuytren disease. J Hand Surg Am 2012;37(9):1820–3.
6. Vlot MAW, PM. Effectiveness of percutaneous needle fasciotomy for second or higher recurrence in Dupuytren contracture. In: Werker PMDJE, Reichert C, Wach B, et al, editors. Duputren disease and related diseases: the cutting edge. Switzerland: Springer; 2017. p. 179–84.
7. Popovic D, Gan BS, Grewal R. Traversing the neurovascular bundle at the level of the metacarpophalangeal joint in palmar fasciectomy for Dupuytren disease. J Hand Surg Am 2012;37(3):626–7.
8. Chen NC, Srinivasan RC, Shauver MJ, et al. A systematic review of outcomes of fasciotomy, aponeurotomy, and collagenase treatments for Dupuytren's contracture. Hand (N Y) 2011;6(3):250–5.
9. Bear BJ, Peimer CA, Kaplan FTD, et al. Treatment of recurrent dupuytren contracture in joints previously effectively treated with collagenase Clostridium histolyticum. J Hand Surg Am 2017;42(5):391.e1-e8.
10. Swanson JW, Watt AJ, Vedder NB. Skin graft loss resulting from collagenase Clostridium histolyticum treatment of Dupuytren contracture: case report and review of the literature. J Hand Surg Am 2013;38(3):548–51.
11. Denkler K. Collagenase for recurrent Dupuytren contracture with skin grafts. J Hand Surg Am 2013;38(6):1264.
12. Skirven TM, Bachoura A, Jacoby SM, et al. The effect of a therapy protocol for increasing correction of severely contracted proximal interphalangeal joints caused by Dupuytren disease and treated with collagenase injection. J Hand Surg Am 2013;38(4):684–9.
13. Peimer CA, Wilbrand S, Gerber RA, et al. Safety and tolerability of collagenase Clostridium histolyticum and fasciectomy for Dupuytren's contracture. J Hand Surg Eur Vol 2015;40(2):141–9.

14. Peimer CA, McGoldrick CA, Kaufman G. Nonsurgical treatment of Dupuytren contracture: 3-year safety results using collagenase *Clostridium histolyticum*. J Hand Surg 2013;38(10):e52.

15. Konneker S, Broelsch GF, Krezdorn N, et al. Multiple recurrences in aggressive forms of Dupuytren's disease: can patients benefit from repeated selective fasciectomy? Plast Reconstr Surg Glob Open 2017;5(2):e1247.

16. Spies CK, Hahn P, Muller LP, et al. The efficacy of open partial aponeurectomy for recurrent Dupuytren's contracture. Arch Orthop Trauma Surg 2016; 136(6):881–9.

17. Bulstrode NW, Jemec B, Smith PJ. The complications of Dupuytren's contracture surgery. J Hand Surg Am 2005;30(5):1021–5.

18. Roush TF, Stern PJ. Results following surgery for recurrent Dupuytren's disease. J Hand Surg Am 2000;25(2):291–6.

19. Sennwald GR. Fasciectomy for treatment of Dupuytren's disease and early complications. J Hand Surg Am 1990;15(5):755–61.

20. Denkler K. Surgical complications associated with fasciectomy for Dupuytren's disease: a 20-year review of the English literature. Eplasty 2010;10:e15.

21. Tonkin MA, Burke FD, Varian JP. Dupuytren's contracture: a comparative study of fasciectomy and dermofasciectomy in one hundred patients. J Hand Surg Br 1984;9(2):156–62.

22. Hueston JT. The control of recurrent Dupuytren's contracture by skin replacement. Br J Plast Surg 1969;22(2):152–6.

23. Brotherston TM, Balakrishnan C, Milner RH, et al. Long term follow-up of dermofasciectomy for Dupuytren's contracture. Br J Plast Surg 1994;47(6): 440–3.

24. Armstrong JR, Hurren JS, Logan AM. Dermofasciectomy in the management of Dupuytren's disease. J Bone Joint Surg Br 2000;82(1):90–4.

25. Chen W, Zhou H, Pan ZJ, et al. The role of skin and subcutaneous tissues in Dupuytren's contracture: an electron microscopic observation. Orthop Surg 2009;1(3):216–21.

26. Villani F, Choughri H, Pelissier P. Importance of skin graft in preventing recurrence of Dupuytren's contracture. Chir Main 2009;28(6):349–51 [in French].

27. Ullah AS, Dias JJ, Bhowal B. Does a 'firebreak' full-thickness skin graft prevent recurrence after surgery for Dupuytren's contracture? A prospective, randomised trial. J Bone Joint Surg Br 2009;91(3):374–8.

28. Tubiana R. Dupuytren's disease of the radial side of the hand. Hand Clin 1999;15(1):149–59.

29. Jones NF, Huang JI. Emergency microsurgical revascularization for critical ischemia during surgery for Dupuytren's contracture: a case report. J Hand Surg Am 2001;26(6):1125–8.

30. Messina A. The TEC (continuous elongation technique) in Dupuytren's disease with serious retraction of the fingers: from amputation to reconstruction. Chir Della Mano 1989;26:253–7.

31. Bailey AJ, Tarlton JF, Van der Stappen J, et al. The continuous elongation technique for severe Dupuytren's disease. A biochemical mechanism. J Hand Surg Br 1994;19(4):522–7.

32. Citron N, Messina JC. The use of skeletal traction in the treatment of severe primary Dupuytren's disease. J Bone Joint Surg Br 1998;80(1):126–9.

33. Messina JC, Messina A. Indications of the continuous extension technique (TEC) for severe Dupuyten disease and recurrences. In: Werker PMDJE, Reichert C, Wach B, et al, editors. Dupuytren disease and related diseases: the cutting edge. Switzerland: Springer; 2017. p. 311–6.

34. Craft RO, Smith AA, Coakley B, et al. Preliminary soft-tissue distraction versus checkrein ligament release after fasciectomy in the treatment of Dupuytren proximal interphalangeal joint contractures. Plast Reconstr Surg 2011;128(5):1107–13.

35. White JW, Kang SN, Nancoo T, et al. Management of severe Dupuytren's contracture of the proximal interphalangeal joint with use of a central slip facilitation device. J Hand Surg Eur Vol 2012;37(8):728–32.

Advances in Minimally Invasive Treatment of Dupuytren Disease

Steven E.R. Hovius, MD, PhD[a,b,c,*], Chao Zhou, MD[b,d]

KEYWORDS

- Dupuytren disease • Fat grafting • Lipofilling • Minimally invasive • Needle fasciotomy
- Needle aponeurotomy • Fasciectomy • Dermofasciectomy

KEY POINTS

- Comparison is provided between minimally invasive techniques (including collagenase) and limited fasciectomy (LF) in the treatment of Dupuytren disease (DD).
- Percutaneous needle aponeurotomy and lipofilling (PALF) is a novel strategy in the treatment of DD.
- There is no difference in contracture correction and recurrent contractures within 1 year when PALF is compared with LF.
- At 5 years' follow-up, LF has significantly less recurrence compared with PALF.
- Often the choice for a patient with moderate Dupuytren diathesis is between early recurrence, fast recovery, and few complications versus late recurrence, slower recovery, and more complications.

INTRODUCTION

Dupuytren disease (DD) is a chronic progressive fibroproliferative disease originating at the palmar fascia. Due to the intricate relationship of fascia with the overlying skin, however, it could be better characterized as a fascia-skin disease. Clinically, DD starts with nodules and pits on the palmar side of the hand. Nodules or thickened areas can also form on the dorsal side at the PIP joints (Garrod pads). Subsequently, cords can develop into flexion contractures of the digits, especially at the MCP and PIP joints.[1] These contractures range from mild contractures that hardly hamper hand function to severe debilitating contractures. Typical activities during daily life that become troublesome to patients include shaking hands, washing their face, wearing gloves, and reaching for objects in narrow spaces.

The disease is more prevalent in the northern part of Europe. Men are more affected than woman, and it occurs more frequently in older patients.[2,3] Genetic research has displayed genetic pathways and subsequently family predisposition for DD.[4] Prevalence varies considerably from 0.2% to 25% depending on country and inclusion criteria.[5]

Previous reported risk factors for DD include trauma, vibrating forces, and diseases like diabetes and epilepsy as well as intoxicating agents like alcohol consumption and smoking.[5–7]

The diathesis or severity of the disease in patients is important. In the moderate diathesis, patients are typically in their sixth decade, and the disease starts in a majority of cases in the ring and/or small finger. In patients with severe diathesis, every ray may be affected. In these patients there is typically:

1. Bilateral hand involvement
2. Ectopic disease
3. Early onset of the disease

[a] Department of Plastic, Reconstructive and Hand Surgery, Erasmus MC, s Gravendijkwal 230, Rotterdam 3015 CE, The Netherlands; [b] Hand and Wrist Surgery, Xpert Clinic, Rotterdam, The Netherlands; [c] Department of Plastic Surgery, Radboudumc, Nijmegen, The Netherlands; [d] Department of Plastic and Reconstructive Surgery, Maastricht University Medical Center, Maastricht, The Netherlands
* Corresponding author. s Gravendijkwal 230, Rotterdam 3015 CE, The Netherlands.
E-mail address: s.e.r.hovius@erasmusmc.nl

Hand Clin 34 (2018) 417–426
https://doi.org/10.1016/j.hcl.2018.03.010
0749-0712/18/© 2018 Elsevier Inc. All rights reserved.

4. A positive family history of DD[8]

Severe diathesis is associated with a higher incidence of recurrent disease after treatment.[1,8]

PATHOPHYSIOLOGY

The exact mechanism underlying the trigger to form nodules and cords at a later age is not fully understood. Millesi[9] holds the view that cellular proliferation is preceded by fibrosis of existing collagen fibers. The pathology starts with changes in the viscoelastic properties of the palmar fascia. The trigger could be the longitudinal stress of the fibers due to incomplete relaxation, which then stimulates the formation of collagen, leading to fibrosis.[9] Mechanical stress seems important, because myofibroblasts disappear in the late stages of DD when the tension is released by operation.[10]

Gabbiani and Majno[11] depicted the role of the conversion of fibroblasts in the palmar area in DD into active myofibroblasts causing contractile forces. Myofibroblasts characteristically express α-smooth muscle actin, which is the actin isoform typical of vascular smooth muscle cells and is important in wound contraction.[12] The conversion can be caused by different environmental factors, including exposure to a variety of different growth factors and cytokines, cell-to-cell interactions, and high extracellular stress from the mechanical properties of the extracellular matrix.[13]

These densely packed myofibroblasts, next to the extracellular matrix, are very active in the nodules in the palm of the hand and fingers, give rise to pits and contracted skin, and eventually mature into cords.[14] In the active nodules, collagen type 1 is converted into type 3, which resembles scar tissue. Cords contain far fewer myofibroblasts and are nearly acellular.[15,16] In DD, the myofibroblast expression is persistent, in contrast to ordinary scar tissue.[17] The myofibroblast in DD is 30% less mobile than in normal palmar fascia; this reduced migration gives rise to mature focal adhesions, which exert greater stress with consequent development of fibrosis.[18,19] The fibrotic process is complex and still not fully understood. The only way to develop new strategies is through improved understanding of the underlying pathophysiologic processes.

TREATMENT

DD is a chronic and progressive disease. Because no curative treatment exists, the primary treatment goals remain to fully straighten the affected ray(s) with a short convalescence period, while reducing the risk of recurrence and avoiding complications.

Treatment options vary widely for DD. Currently there is a jungle of treatment possibilities out there, often without any physiologic background. Indications for treatment are flexion contractures of MCP joints and/or PIP joints. Often 30° is used as a parameter; however, this threshold is not an exact science and should be adjusted depending on the individual needs, impairment, and expectations of the patient.

Nonsurgical treatment includes splinting, medication, and radiotherapy. There is no evidence that splinting alone can prevent the development of contractures. Medication is beyond the scope of this article, but is discussed in more detail in Paul M.N. Werker and Ilse Degreef's article, "Alternative and Adjunctive Treatments for Dupuytren Disease," in this issue. Radiotherapy has been used in DD in the early stages to prevent or delay further progression.[20,21] Results in the literature are variable, with some showing no difference compared with controls and others reporting a delay in the development of contractures in the irradiated group.[22,23]

More invasive treatment can consist of interrupting the cord with or without interposition of a skin graft or other biomaterial or attempting to remove as much as pathologic tissue as possible, also with or without the use of skin graft or even flaps. Four guiding theories underlie this. The first is to treat the cord very locally. The second is trying to excise the cord partially and inserting a full-thickness skin graft or a cellulose implant with the idea of creating a fire break. A third approach is fully excising all pathologic tissue, much akin to treating a tumor. A fourth approach is combining extensive surgery with a skin graft or flap with the assumption that recurrence rarely, if ever, comes back under the graft. When considering these approaches, it is important to take into consideration the diathesis of the patient and whether it is a primary or secondary case. Comparisons of long-term outcomes of the different approaches is hardly possible, because of different definitions for outcomes, such as recurrence, across the studies describing each technique. Nevertheless, there are certainly trends that can be detected looking at the published literature.

The most commonly used surgical procedure remains limited fasciectomy (LF) with primary closure. This has not changed for decades. Assessed after a minimum of 5 years' follow-up, reported recurrence rates range from 20.9% to 46.5%.[24,25] Complications after LF include edema, hematoma, infection, paresthesias, neurovascular injuries, pain, tendon ruptures, and complex regional pain syndrome (CRPS). In a previously published randomized controlled trial (RCT), the overall cumulative complication rate for LF was 30%.[26]

If primary closure is not possible, or not preferred, the palm may be partly left open according to the McCash method. Reported 5-year recurrence rate was 41% with 23% of the patients having a severe diathesis. Early age of onset, major involvement of the PIP joint, and localization at the fifth ray predisposed to developing recurrence in this study. Early complications, such as hematoma, skin necrosis, or infection, were not reported using the McCash method.[27,28]

More extensive surgical procedures involving the use of full-thickness skin grafts were introduced many decades ago and deemed particularly appropriate in patients with recurrent disease and/or severe diathesis. Many investigators have demonstrated that disease recurrence rarely occurs underneath the skin grafts with reported rates of 0% to 8.4% assessed up to 6 years after treatment. The best results were obtained when the grafts were extended to the midlateral line on both sides of the digits to prevent disease extension from developing into contractures at the edges of the grafts. A low incidence of disease extension was also reported (9%). Complications were, however, more common than in LF, which included hematoma, loss of skin graft, infection, and neurovascular damage.[25,29–32] Ullah and colleagues[33] published a RCT comparing fasciectomy with and without full-thickness skin grafts at the PIP joint and found no difference between treatment groups with a recurrence rate of 12.2% after 3 years' follow-up.

In highly selected cases of severe recurrent disease with a prior history of multiple surgeries, the first author (S.E.R.H) has used pedicled arm flaps to cover the palm of the hand, including the proximal phalanx of all fingers as a replacement of the diseased fascia and skin. No disease recurrence was found underneath the flap even after more than 20 years.[34]

The trend toward less invasive surgery probably started with Moermans'[35] segmental fasciectomy, in which cords are partially removed at different levels in a stepwise fashion. The investigators reported fewer complications and faster recovery than traditional LF. In a prospective study involving severe diathesis cases, Degreef and colleagues[7] assessed segmental fasciectomy with and without the use of an absorbable cellulose sheet. The group in which a cellulose sheet was inserted had 87% correction versus 51% in the group without the sheet. With the implant, range of movement improved significantly (by 33%), which remained unchanged through 1 year follow-up.

MINIMALLY INVASIVE TECHNIQUES

In the past 2 decades, there has been an increase in popularity of minimally invasive techniques, in part due to the long recovery period after LF, especially after reoperations. The most recent addition is injectable collagenase *Clostridium histolyticum* (CCH), which selectively disintegrates collagen. The technique involves the injection of a small volume of collagenase solution into the pathologic cord(s), thus weakening the treated areas to allow for subsequent rupture by manipulation of the contracted finger. CCH has been popularized by Hurst and colleagues since 2000. Clinical success rates (defined as correction of contracture to 0°–5° from full extension) have been reported to be as high as 87%. Two-year recurrence rates have been reported at 19%. Adverse events are common but are almost always local and transient. Although tendon ruptures and CRPS have been described, they occur rarely.[36,37] At 5-year follow-up, the overall recurrence rate for successful treatment with CCH was 47%: 39% at the MCP joint and 66% at the PIP joint. Skin atrophy was observed as a long-term complication in 1 patient.[38] Skov and colleagues[39] reported 83% recurrence at 2-year follow-up after CCH treatment. After a free trial in the Netherlands, CCH is currently not reimbursed.

Perhaps the most accepted minimally invasive technique is percutaneous needle fasciotomy (PNF). It is interesting that Baron Guillaume de Dupuytren (1834), after which the disease is named, cut the cord in the palmar fascia, thus performing a fasciotomy. Henry Cline, however, probably preceded Dupuytren by performing the first fasciotomy in 1808.[40] It took more than 200 years to return to less invasive methods in a more sophisticated way; needle fasciotomy was introduced by the French rheumatologist Lermusiaux in 1980 and brought to the hand surgeons by Foucher in 2003. In Foucher and colleagues' series,[41] the postoperative gain was prominent at the MCP level: 79% versus 65% at interphalangeal level. The reoperation rate was 24%. In the group assessed at 3.2 years' follow-up, the recurrence rate was 58%, and disease "activity" was 69%. The convalescence period was short, and only 1 nerve was damaged in a recurrent case.[41]

van Rijssen and colleagues[24] reported 63% contracture reduction after PNF in an RCT. The recurrence rate was 65% after 3 years and 85% after 5 years.

Table 1 summarizes the results of recent studies that have directly compared CCH, PNF, and LF in terms of their outcomes.[39,42–49] Placebo-controlled studies or those describing a

Table 1
Summary of the results of recent studies that have directly compared the outcomes of collagenase *Clostridium histolyticum*, percutaneous needle fasciotomy, and limited fasciectomy

Authors, Year[a]	Treatments Compared	Setting (Country)	Study Design	No. Patients	Contracture Correction	Complications/Adverse Events	Long-Term Outcomes
Atroshi et al,[42] 2014	CCH vs LF	Single center (Sweden)	Retrospective cohort	32	CCH 20° vs LF 19° mean residual total extension deficit at 5–6 wk post-treatment	No complications observed	NA
Kan et al,[43] 2016	PALF vs LF	Multicenter (NL)	RCT	80	For MCP joints and PIP joints no significant difference in contracture correction between both treatment groups (no exact values are reported)	PALF 5% vs LF 9% complications through 1 y, NS	PALF 18% vs LF 9% recurrence at 1 y, NS
Naam,[44] 2013	CCH vs fasciectomy	Single center (US)	Retrospective cohort	46	For MCP contractures, CCH 3.6° vs LF 3.7° at average 32 mo, NS. For PIP contracture, CCH 17.5° vs LF 8.1° at average 32 mo, NS	No statistical comparison provided.	NA
Nydick et al,[45] 2013	CCH vs PNA	Single center (US)	Retrospective cohort	59	CCH 56% vs PNA 67% reduction of contracture within 0–5 of normal at mean 6-mo, NS	No statistical comparison provided	NA
Scherman et al,[46] 2016	PNA vs CCH	Multicenter (Sweden)	RCT	93	PNA 75% vs CCH 75% reduction in contracture at 1 y, NS	No statistical comparison provided	NA

Skov et al,[39] 2017	CCH vs PNA	Multicenter (Denmark)	RCT	50	CCH 7% vs PNA 29% maintained clinical improvement at 2 y (a reduction in contracture of >50% from baseline), NS	CCH 93% vs PNA 24% transient complications, $P<.05$	CCH 83% vs PNA 68% recurrence at 2 y, NS
Strömberg et al,[47] 2016	CCH vs PNA	Multicenter (Sweden)	RCT	140	CCH 88% vs PNA 90% correction to <5° at 1 y, NS.	No statistical comparison provided	NA
Zhou et al,[48] 2015	CCH vs LF	Multicenter (NL)	Prospective cohort	132	For affected MCP joints, CCH 13° vs LF 6° residual contracture at 6–12 wk, NS. For affected PIP joints, CCH 25° vs 15° residual contracture at 6–12 wk, $P = .010$	CCH 0/66 cases vs LF 4/66 serious AEs, $P = .042$	NA
Zhou et al,[49] 2017	CCH vs PNA	Multicenter (NL)	Prospective cohort	130	For affected MCP joints, CCH 71% vs PNA 65% reduction from baseline at 6–12 wk, NS. For affected PIP joints, CCH 42% vs PNA 50% reduction from baseline at 6–12 wk, NS	Incidence of AEs that occurred after both treatments (sensory disturbance and skin fissures) was similar.	NA

Abbreviations: AE, adverse event; N, null; NA, not assessed; NL, the Netherlands; NS, not statistically significant; PNA, percutaneous needle aponeurotomy or asciotomy.
[a] Alphabetical order. First author is reported.

single technique were not included because the results of such studies cannot be validly compared as a result of differences in patient selection, definition of outcomes, and follow-up time points.

In an attempt to reduce the high recurrence rates in PNF, the authors searched for new strategies to prevent fibrosis. One of these strategies uses adipose-derived stem cells (ADSCs), which have been used effectively to treat other fibrotic diseases.[50–53] The effect of ADSCs on myofibroblast activity has been investigated by the authors' group. In 1 of the studies, these stem cells were shown to inhibit proliferation of the contractile myofibroblasts and mediate these effects by soluble factors, influenced by cell contact[54] (**Fig. 1**). Because lipoaspirates are known to be a rich source of ADSCs with regenerative potential, the authors aimed to use a lipoaspirate after contracture release in DD.[55–57]

Subdermal fat deficiency and atrophy occurs in DD as pathologic fibrosis displaces the fat.[58] Therefore, autologous fat grafting seems logical as an adjunct to restore this fat loss not only as padding but also to promote wound healing. Flexion contractures of the digits have already been infiltrated with fat in the diseased area in the early twentieth century as a treatment of DD.[59] The authors reintroduced this procedure, because autologous fat grafting has seen an increase in popularity over the past decade for a variety of conditions and diseases. Because conventional open surgery requires extensive dissection of every ray through multiple stages, the great advantage of this technique is its ability to treat multiray disease in a single session (**Figs. 2** and **3**).

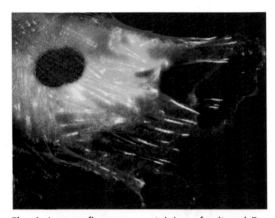

Fig. 1. Immunofluorescence staining of cultured Dupuytren myofibroblast. (*From* Hovius S, Verhoekx J, Kan H, et al. Lipo-filling as a new treatment strategy for Dupuytren's disease: from basic science to clinical results. In: Warwick D, editor. Dupuytren's disease FESSH instructional course 2015. Torino (Italy): C. G. Edizioni Medico Scientifiche s.r.l.; 2015. p. 198; with permission.)

Long-standing PIP joint contractures are not easily completely released by this technique due to inherent joint contracture and attenuation of the extensor tendon central slip. The authors advise against treatment of patients who have received flaps in the affected area, because the scarred neurovascular bundles are no longer loose and, therefore, at risk for injury.

Compared with the traditional PNF, the authors made 2 important adaptations. First, the needle technique is different. The authors use an extensive percutaneous needle aponeurotomy technique with multiple superficial nicks over the cord and nodules over a distance of 1 mm to 2 mm along the whole ray. The affected ray is continuously under tension, which brings the cord more palmarly, thereby lowering the risk of injuring the neurovascular bundle. When the finger is stretched, the overlying treated palmar skin is then loosened in the subcutaneous layer to create a scaffold that is permissive to the grafted fat. Second, the grafted fat, typically obtained from the abdomen or inner thighs by liposuction, is not centrifuged. As soon as the fat layers have settled by gravity, the lipoaspirate is diffusely injected through 2 to 3 needle entry sites in the palm and the digit. Typically, a total of 10-mL lipoaspirate per ray is injected. After bandaging, a plaster splint is applied with the fingers extended for not more than a week, followed by hand therapy and a night splint for 3 months. The authors have named this new technique percutaneous aponeurotomy and lipofilling (PALF).[60–62]

The authors have conducted an RCT comparing 40 patients treated with the PALF technique with 40 patients undergoing LF. The outcome measures we used in the RCT included patient satisfaction, convalescence period, and objective measurements of range of motion and contracture recurrence. The PALF technique demonstrates a significantly shorter convalescence and similar operative contracture correction compared with LF. The MCP joints were fully corrected, whereas the PIP joints had a residual contracture. After 1 year, no significant differences in results were found with LF; recurrence was 18% for the joints treated with PALF and 9% for the LF treated group. The definition used for recurrence was an increase of contracture of at least 20° at 1 year post-treatment compared with 3 weeks post-treatment. Furthermore, a lower incidence of long-term complications were encountered in the PALF group.[43]

At 5 years, however, the long-term results favored LF, with 74% recurrence in the PALF group versus 39% in the LF group when considering affected MCP and PIP joints. These

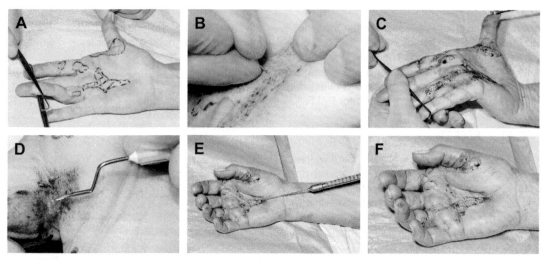

Fig. 2. The PALF procedure. (*A*) Perioperative photograph showing marked area of the affected tissue. (*B*) Release of the cord by multiple punctures with a 19-gauge needle. (*C*) Fully released contracture and straightening of the fingers. (*D*) An angled needle is used to release the skin further from the underlying subcutaneous tissue. (*E*) Lipofilling of the operated area. (*F*) Slight ballooning of the palmar skin. (*From* Hovius S, Verhoekx J, Kan H, et al. Lipofilling as a new treatment strategy for Dupuytren's disease: from basic science to clinical results. Section 4.7 page 201 and 202. In: Warwick D, editor. Dupuytren's disease FESSH instructional course 2015. Torino (Italy): C. G. Edizioni Med-ico Scientifiche s.r.l.; 2015; with permission.)

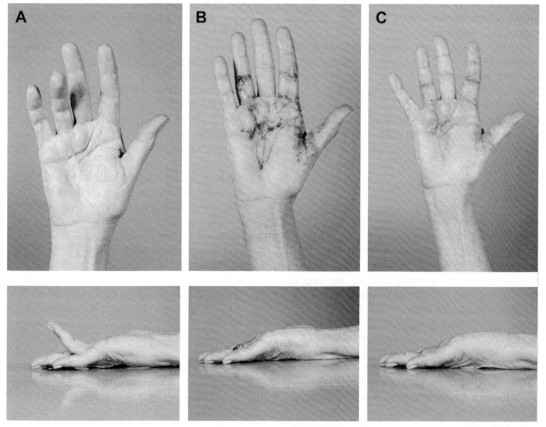

Fig. 3. A clinical case treated with the PALF procedure. (*A*) Perioperative photograph showing a primary Dupuytren contracture; (*B*) 2-week postoperative photographs; and (*C*) 6-month postoperative photographs. (*From* Hovius S, Verhoekx J, Kan H, et al. Lipofilling as a new treatment strategy for Dupuytren's disease: from basic science to clinical results. Section 4.7 page 201 and 202. In: Warwick D, editor. Dupuytren's disease FESSH instructional course 2015. Torino (Italy): C. G. Edizioni Med-ico Scientifiche s.r.l.; 2015; with permission.)

long-term results for PALF seem better than those reported previously for traditional PNF but were not as good as expected. Therefore, the authors believe that patients who prefer a more rapid recovery and lower risk of complications over lower risk of recurrence to be more suited for PALF.

FUTURE PERSPECTIVES

In any chronic disease for which no curative treatment exists, the ultimate goal is a noninvasive drug or therapy with minimal side effects. Perhaps the most illustrative example of how advances in medical therapy have made surgery almost obsolete is the advent of biologicals for the treatment of rheumatoid arthritis patients. Maybe someday, a similar situation might occur for DD. The authors believe, however, that CCH is not going to be that biological, although it has changed the practice of hand surgeons tremendously in countries where insurers do reimburse the treatment. Trials in DD with other medications, like anti–tissue necrosis factor, are ongoing. The complex pathway of fibrosis formation is, however, a cascade of events, which implies that DD will not easily be treated by a single drug.

Luckily, many basic research studies are currently under way, gradually advancing understanding in these areas. The vast amount of recent studies on DD demonstrate that this is an era of increased options and interest in DD. The authors, therefore, believe that the quest to improve treatment of DD will continue to attract and challenge clinicians and surgeons alike worldwide.

SUMMARY

In the past 200 years, the treatment of DD, a chronic fibroproliferative disease of the palmar fascia and skin, has evolved from simple fasciotomy of a cord to extensive surgical options, only to return again to minimally invasive techniques, such as PNF and collagenase injection.

A novel technique called PALF is described. In an RCT, no difference was found between the recurrence rates of PALF compared with LF at 1 year follow-up; however, at 5 years, there were significantly more recurrences in the PALF group.

Therefore, patients with a moderate diathesis should make a shared decision with a caregiver to choose either a minimally invasive technique with potential for early recurrence but faster recovery and fewer complications versus a more invasive option like LF or dermofasciectomy with less recurrence but slower recovery and more complications. In patients with multiple recurrences and

severe diathesis, the choice for minimal invasive techniques may be less advisable.

REFERENCES

1. McFarlane R, McGrouther DA, Flint MH. Dupuytren's disease. Edinburgh (Scotland): Churchill Livingstone; 1990.
2. Lanting R, van den Heuvel ER, Westerink B, et al. Prevalence of dupuytren disease in The Netherlands. Plast Reconstr Surg 2013;132(2):394–403.
3. Mikkelsen OA. The prevalence of Dupuytren's disease in Norway. A study in a representative population sample of the municipality of Haugesund. Acta Chir Scand 1972;138(7):695–700.
4. Dolmans GH, Werker PM, Hennies HC, et al. Wnt signaling and Dupuytren's disease. N Engl J Med 2011;365(4):307–17.
5. Lanting R, Broekstra DC, Werker PM, et al. A systematic review and meta-analysis on the prevalence of Dupuytren disease in the general population of Western countries. Plast Reconstr Surg 2014; 133(3):593–603.
6. Geoghegan JM, Forbes J, Clark DI, et al. Dupuytren's disease risk factors. J Hand Surg Br 2004; 29(5):423–6.
7. Degreef I, Tejpar S, De Smet L. Postoperative outcome of segmental fasciectomy in Dupuytren's Disease improves by creating firebreaks with an absorbable cellulose implant. J Plast Surg Hand Surg 2011;45(3):26–300.
8. Abe Y, Rokkaku T, Ofuchi S, et al. An objective method to evaluate the risk of recurrence and extension of Dupuytren's disease. J Hand Surg Br 2004; 29(5):427–30.
9. Millesi H. On the pathogenesis and therapy of Dupuytren's contracture. (A study based on more than 500 cases). Ergeb Chir Orthop 1965;47:51–101 [in German].
10. Gabbiani G. The myofibroblast in wound healing and fibrocontractive diseases. J Pathol 2003; 200(4):500–3.
11. Gabbiani G, Majno G. Dupuytren's contracture: fibroblast contraction? An ultrastructural study. Am J Pathol 1972;66(1):131–46.
12. Skalli O, Ropraz P, Trzeciak A, et al. A monoclonal antibody against alpha-smooth muscle actin: a new probe for smooth muscle differentiation. J Cell Biol 1986;103(6 Pt 2):2787–96.
13. Hinz B. Formation and function of the myofibroblast during tissue repair. J Invest Dermatol 2007;127(3): 526–37.
14. Luck JV. Dupuytren's contracture; a new concept of the pathogenesis correlated with surgical management. J Bone Joint Surg Am 1959;41-A(4):635–64.
15. Verjee LS, Midwood K, Davidson D, et al. Myofibroblast distribution in Dupuytren's cords: correlation

with digital contracture. J Hand Surg Am 2009; 34(10):1785–94.

16. McFarlane RM. Patterns of the diseased fascia in the fingers in Dupuytren's contracture. Displacement of the neurovascular bundle. Plast Reconstr Surg 1974;54(1):31–44.

17. Darby I, Skalli O, Gabbiani G. Alpha-smooth muscle actin is transiently expressed by myofibroblasts during experimental wound healing. Lab Invest 1990; 63(1):21–9.

18. Tomasek JJ, Gabbiani G, Hinz B, et al. Myofibroblasts and mechano-regulation of connective tissue remodelling. Nat Rev Mol Cell Biol 2002;3(5):349–63.

19. Goffin JM, Pittet P, Csucs G, et al. Focal adhesion size controls tension-dependent recruitment of alpha-smooth muscle actin to stress fibers. J Cell Biol 2006;172(2):259–68.

20. Seegenschmiedt MH, Olschewski T, Guntrum F. Optimization of radiotherapy in Dupuytren's disease. Initial results of a controlled trial. Strahlenther Onkol 2001;177(2):74–81 [in German].

21. Betz N, Ott OJ, Adamietz B, et al. Radiotherapy in early-stage Dupuytren's contracture. Long-term results after 13 years. Strahlenther Onkol 2010; 186(2):82–90.

22. Seegenschmiedt MH, Keilholz L, Wielputz M, et al. Long-term outcome of radiotherapy for early stage dupuytren's disease: a phase III clinical study. Berlin: Springer-Verlag Berlin Heidelberg; 2012.

23. Weinzierl G, Flugel M, Geldmacher J. Lack of effectiveness of alternative non-surgical treatment procedures of Dupuytren contracture. Chirurg 1993; 64(6):492–4 [in German].

24. van Rijssen AL, ter Linden H, Werker PM. Five-year results of a randomized clinical trial on treatment in Dupuytren's disease: percutaneous needle fasciotomy versus limited fasciectomy. Plast Reconstr Surg 2012;129(2):469–77.

25. Tonkin MA, Burke FD, Varian JP. Dupuytren's contracture: a comparative study of fasciectomy and dermofasciectomy in one hundred patients. J Hand Surg Br 1984;9(2):156–62.

26. van Rijssen AL, Gerbrandy FS, Ter Linden H, et al. A comparison of the direct outcomes of percutaneous needle fasciotomy and limited fasciectomy for Dupuytren's disease: a 6-week follow-up study. J Hand Surg Am 2006;31(5):717–25.

27. McCash CR. The open palm technique in dupuytren's contracture. Br J Plast Surg 1964;17:271–80.

28. Foucher G, Cornil C, Lenoble E. "Open palm" technique in Dupuytren's disease. Postoperative complications and results after more than 5 years. Chirurgie 1992;118(4):189–94 [discussion: 195–6]. [in French].

29. Hueston JT. Digital wolfe grafts in recurrent Dupuytren's contracture. Plast Reconstr Surg Transplant Bull 1962;29:342–4.

30. Ketchum LD, Hixson FP. Dermofasciectomy and full-thickness grafts in the treatment of Dupuytren's contracture. J Hand Surg Am 1987;12(5 Pt 1):659–64.

31. Hall PN, Fitzgerald A, Sterne GD, et al. Skin replacement in Dupuytren's disease. J Hand Surg Br 1997; 22(2):193–7.

32. Armstrong JR, Hurren JS, Logan AM. Dermofasciectomy in the management of Dupuytren's disease. J Bone Joint Surg Br 2000;82(1):90–4.

33. Ullah AS, Dias JJ, Bhowal B. Does a 'firebreak' full-thickness skin graft prevent recurrence after surgery for Dupuytren's contracture?: a prospective, randomised trial. J Bone Joint Surg Br 2009;91(3):374–8.

34. Kan HJ, Hovius SE. Long-term follow-up of flaps for extensive Dupuytren's and Ledderhose disease in one family. J Plast Reconstr Aesthet Surg 2012; 65(12):1741–5.

35. Moermans JP. Long-term results after segmental aponeurectomy for Dupuytren's disease. J Hand Surg Br 1996;21(6):797–800.

36. Hurst LC, Badalamente MA, Hentz VR, et al. Injectable collagenase clostridium histolyticum for Dupuytren's contracture. N Engl J Med 2009;361(10): 968–79.

37. Watt AJ, Curtin CM, Hentz VR. Collagenase injection as nonsurgical treatment of Dupuytren's disease: 8-year follow-up. J Hand Surg Am 2010;35(4):534–9, 539.e1.

38. Peimer CA, Blazar P, Coleman S, et al. Dupuytren contracture recurrence following treatment with collagenase clostridium histolyticum (CORDLESS [Collagenase Option for Reduction of Dupuytren Long-Term Evaluation of Safety Study]): 5-year data. J Hand Surg Am 2015;40(8):1597–605.

39. Skov ST, Bisgaard T, Sondergaard P, et al. Injectable collagenase versus percutaneous needle fasciotomy for Dupuytren contracture in proximal interphalangeal joints: a randomized controlled trial. J Hand Surg Am 2017;42(5):321–8.e3.

40. Elliot D. The early history of contracture of the palmar fascia. Part 1: the origin of the disease: the curse of the MacCrimmons: the hand of benediction: Cline's contracture. J Hand Surg Br 1988; 13(3):246–53.

41. Foucher G, Medina J, Navarro R. Percutaneous needle aponeurotomy: complications and results. J Hand Surg Br 2003;28(5):427–31.

42. Atroshi I, Strandberg E, Lauritzson A, et al. Costs for collagenase injections compared with fasciectomy in the treatment of Dupuytren's contracture: a retrospective cohort study. BMJ Open 2014;4(1): e004166.

43. Kan HJ, Selles RW, van Nieuwenhoven CA, et al. Percutaneous Aponeurotomy and Lipofilling (PALF) versus limited fasciectomy in patients with primary dupuytren's contracture: a prospective, randomized,

controlled trial. Plast Reconstr Surg 2016;137(6): 1800–12.

44. Naam NH. Functional outcome of collagenase injections compared with fasciectomy in treatment of Dupuytren's contracture. Hand (N Y) 2013;8(4):410–6.

45. Nydick JA, Olliff BW, Garcia MJ, et al. A comparison of percutaneous needle fasciotomy and collagenase injection for dupuytren disease. J Hand Surg Am 2013;38(12):2377–80.

46. Scherman P, Jenmalm P, Dahlin LB. One-year results of needle fasciotomy and collagenase injection in treatment of Dupuytren's contracture: a two-centre prospective randomized clinical trial. J Hand Surg Eur Vol 2016;41(6):577–82.

47. Strömberg J, Ibsen-Sorensen A, Friden J. Comparison of treatment outcome after collagenase and needle fasciotomy for dupuytren contracture: a randomized, single-blinded, clinical trial with a 1-year follow-up. J Hand Surg Am 2016;41(9):873–80.

48. Zhou C, Hovius SE, Slijper HP, et al. Collagenase clostridium histolyticum versus limited fasciectomy for dupuytren's contracture: outcomes from a multicenter propensity score matched study. Plast Reconstr Surg 2015;136(1):87–97.

49. Zhou C, Hovius SER, Pieters AJ, et al. Comparative effectiveness of needle aponeurotomy and collagenase injection for dupuytren's contracture: a multicenter study. Plast Reconstr Surg Glob Open 2017;5(9):e1425.

50. Castiglione F, Hedlund P, Van der Aa F, et al. Intratunical injection of human adipose tissue-derived stem cells prevents fibrosis and is associated with improved erectile function in a rat model of Peyronie's disease. Eur Urol 2013;63(3):551–60.

51. Alfarano C, Roubeix C, Chaaya R, et al. Intraparenchymal injection of bone marrow mesenchymal stem cells reduces kidney fibrosis after ischemia-reperfusion in cyclosporine-immunosuppressed rats. Cell Transplant 2012;21(9):2009–19.

52. Zhao W, Li JJ, Cao DY, et al. Intravenous injection of mesenchymal stem cells is effective in treating liver fibrosis. World J Gastroenterol 2012;18(10): 1048–58.

53. Elnakish MT, Kuppusamy P, Khan M. Stem cell transplantation as a therapy for cardiac fibrosis. J Pathol 2013;229(2):347–54.

54. Verhoekx JS, Mudera V, Walbeehm ET, et al. Adipose-derived stem cells inhibit the contractile myofibroblast in Dupuytren's disease. Plast Reconstr Surg 2013;132(5):1139–48.

55. Zuk PA, Zhu M, Ashjian P, et al. Human adipose tissue is a source of multipotent stem cells. Mol Biol Cell 2002;13(12):4279–95.

56. Aust L, Devlin B, Foster SJ, et al. Yield of human adipose-derived adult stem cells from liposuction aspirates. Cytotherapy 2004;6(1):7–14.

57. Coleman SR. Structural fat grafting: more than a permanent filler. Plast Reconstr Surg 2006;118(3 Suppl):108S–20S.

58. Rayan GM. Clinical presentation and types of Dupuytren's disease. Hand Clin 1999;15(1):87–96, vii.

59. Lexer E. Die frei fetttransplantation. In die Freie Transplantation, Teil 1. Stuttgart: Ferdinand Ecke; 1919.

60. Hovius SE, Kan HJ, Smit X, et al. Extensive percutaneous aponeurotomy and lipografting: a new treatment for Dupuytren disease. Plast Reconstr Surg 2011;128(1):221–8.

61. Hovius SER, VS, Kan HJ, et al. Lipo-filling as a new treatment strategy for Dupuytren's disease. From basic science to clinical results. Dupuytren's Disease, FESSH Instructional Course 2015: Editor in Chief: David Warwick. 2015. p. 197–205.

62. Hovius SER, Kan HJ, Verhoekx JSN, et al. Percutaneous aponeurotomy and lipofilling as a regenerative treatment aleternative for dupuytren's disease. Section six upper extremity [Chapter 44]. In: Coleman SR, Mazzola RF, Lee LQ, et al, editors. Fat injection from filling to regeneration. 2nd edition. New York: Thieme; 2017. ISBN978-1-62623-675-2.

Bringing It All Together
A Practical Approach to the Treatment of Dupuytren Disease

Steven C. Haase, MD*, Kevin C. Chung, MD, MS

KEYWORDS

- Dupuytren disease • Collagenase • Fasciectomy • Shared decision making
- Evidence-based medicine

KEY POINTS

- Interventions for Dupuytren disease range from minimally invasive options (needle aponeurotomy, collagenase injection) to extensive surgeries (fasciectomy, dermofasciectomy).
- Because no option is completely curative, and each has associated risks, decisions about treatment should be made using the best evidence available in a shared decision-making process between the patient and the clinician.
- Regardless of the treatment chosen, a detailed knowledge of anatomy, as well as precise, careful technique, is necessary for the safe, effective, efficient elimination of Dupuytren contractures.

Despite the passage of more than 200 years since Cline first proposed a treatment for Dupuytren disease, debate still continues regarding the optimal intervention for these patients. Even the definition of "optimal" is in flux as one tries to compare techniques based on complexity, effectiveness, cost, and other criteria. Given the worldwide prevalence of Dupuytren disease, one must also consider the implications of the interventions in different cultures, different economies, and different health care delivery systems. It would be quite short-sighted for any practitioner to claim they have developed the "best" algorithm of care, when it is unlikely any one approach will be generalizable to all of the world's populations.

Nonetheless, within the context of a tertiary practice at a high-volume academic medical center, the authors have developed what they believe is a practical approach to the treatment of Dupuytren disease. At its core, it is a *patient-centered approach* heavily based on *shared decision making*: 2 characteristics that should make much of this discussion applicable to a wide range of clinical practices. Their approach begins with a simple assignment of patients into one of 3 groups:

1. Observation (no intervention)
2. Intervention: minimal (clinic based)
3. Intervention: operative (operating room based)

OBSERVATION

Many patients present to the authors' clinic with early Dupuytren disease and require no operative intervention. Some are self-referred, and others are sent by their primary care physician when a new nodule is discovered. A subset of these patients is quite worried about the presence of malignancy, and these patients may require reassurance to help their peace of mind. If patients are unwilling to accept the experienced surgeon's diagnosis, based on history and physical examination, an objective evaluation with ultrasound imaging can confirm the diagnosis at relatively low cost.

Disclosure Statement: The authors have no conflict of interest.
Department of Surgery, Michigan Medicine, University of Michigan Medical School, 2130 Taubman Center, 1500 East Medical Center Drive, Ann Arbor, MI 48109, USA
* Corresponding author.
E-mail address: shaase@med.umich.edu

Hand Clin 34 (2018) 427–436
https://doi.org/10.1016/j.hcl.2018.04.003
0749-0712/18/© 2018 Elsevier Inc. All rights reserved.

hand.theclinics.com

In rare cases, nodules in atypical locations may not be immediately identified as Dupuytren disease by the surgeons, and there is certainly very little morbidity to perform excisional biopsy in these cases. In the authors' experience, postoperative "flares" or worsening of the disease is rare in these patients.

Observation may also be warranted for patients with mild contractures. Despite the appeal of the minimally invasive procedures for this disease, all interventions are accompanied by some risk. Patients with mild proximal interphalangeal (PIP) contractures (less than 30°) that do not interfere with daily function might be considered candidates for surgery in some textbooks. However, in the authors' approach, these patients are carefully evaluated and counseled about their options. A patient with a strong Dupuytren diathesis may recur quickly after operative PIP release, and this can be discouraging for surgeon and patient alike. Even after release of a mild PIP contracture, patients need to be committed to the postoperative therapy program, and they need to understand the chance of recurrence. Many times, after a frank discussion with these patients, the authors decide to take careful measurements of their contractures and reevaluate in 3 to 6 months. If there is demonstrable, objective worsening of the contracture during this period of observation, then both surgeon and patient may feel more comfortable proceeding with an intervention.

INTERVENTION: MINIMAL

In the authors' institution, the demand for collagenase treatment has increased steadily since its US Food and Drug Administration (FDA) approval in 2010. Many patients request this treatment, having been referred by a friend or by their physician specifically for this intervention. Despite the popularity this treatment has achieved, the authors have a detailed discussion about all applicable interventions, ranging from needle aponeurotomy to dermofasciectomy, depending on the patient's needs and presentation.

Patients with distinct cords in the palm leading to metacarpophalangeal (MCP) contractures are excellent candidates for either needle aponeurotomy or collagenase treatment (**Fig. 1**). After educating patients about both treatment options, including the potential costs, risks, and estimated recurrence rates, the authors encourage patients to choose between these interventions freely. Despite telling patients that there is no clear long-term advantage of one over the other, most patients in the authors' institution choose collagenase treatment over needle aponeurotomy.

For palmar cords that extend into the finger, leading to PIP contractures via spiral cords and/or central cords, it is important to evaluate what effect the division/dissolution of the cord will have on the PIP joint. Many of these cords cross both the MCP and the PIP joints (**Fig. 2**). Mobility of the PIP joint is assessed with the MCP flexed, and vice versa, to determine how much of the PIP contracture is attributed to the cord, and how much is intrinsic joint contracture. Although minimally invasive techniques can be used on these distinct cords, one may not expect complete resolution of the PIP contracture if there is intrinsic joint stiffness present. Patients are counseled that they may still have some residual PIP contracture present, even if the palmar cord is completely disrupted by minimally invasive means.

Many patients seek out these minimally invasive treatment options after previously undergoing more invasive surgery. When patients have successfully recovered from fasciectomy, completed all the postoperative therapy, and then develop a recurrence, they are often quite interested in pursuing something less invasive if possible. If distinct

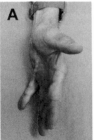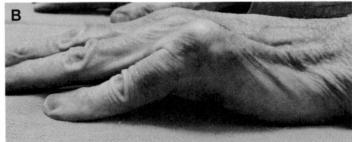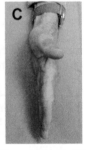

Fig. 1. (*A*) A 73-year-old patient with Dupuytren contracture limited to the MCP joint of the left small finger. (*B*) Failed "table-top test" before collagenase treatment. (*C*) Two months after collagenase treatment, with restoration of full extension.

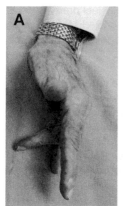 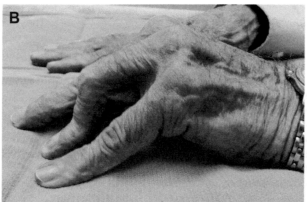 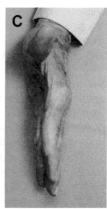

Fig. 2. (*A*) A 79-year-old patient with Dupuytren contracture of the left ring finger, involving both the MCP and the PIP joints. (*B*) "Table-top test." (*C*) Four months after collagenase treatment, with restoration of full extension. Ironically, the patient was wearing the exact same color shirt for the follow-up visit!

cords are identified in the palm, or in the bases of the digits, carefully placed collagenase injections can often give these patients functional improvement without the risk of another big operation.

Given the authors' greater experience with collagenase injection, some of the details of this technique are presented here for the reader's benefit. A more detailed review of needle aponeurotomy technique is presented in Kate E. Elzinga and Michael J. Morhart's article, "Needle Aponeurotomy for Dupuytren Disease," in this issue.

TECHNIQUE: COLLAGENASE INJECTION AND MANIPULATION

The FDA-approved protocol for collagenase injection is available readily online and in the package insert. The comments in later discussion diverge from these recommendations in several ways; the reader is reminded that these modifications are considered an off-label use of the medication.

Patients interested in collagenase injection first must first get authorization for insurance coverage. This step has deterred a couple of patients from this option, because some insurance companies impose steep copayments or deductibles for this expensive medication. Some patients find that their insurance covers the cost of surgery more completely, and they have opted to undergo fasciectomy as a cheaper option.

Once approved, patients are scheduled for 2 clinic visits: one for the injection and one for the manipulation. After performing these interventions on consecutive days for several years, the authors have now gradually shifted to performing them a week apart. This increase in time between injection and manipulation appears to be a growing trend based on feedback

the authors have received from colleagues across the United States. Although it is an off-label protocol, waiting a full week between the injection and the manipulation has anecdotally led to fewer skin tears, while maintaining excellent results overall.

Another modification from the strict FDA-approved protocol is the use of local anesthesia before the collagenase injection. The injection of a small amount of lidocaine into the dermis at the anticipated collagenase injection site or sites has dramatically improved patient comfort and has not led to any measurable decrease in the collagenase's effectiveness in the authors' practice. After injection of lidocaine, the patient is advised to spend 5 to 10 minutes massaging the area, leading to dispersal of the medication and reduction of any local edema/tumescence, allowing the cord to remain easily palpable for the collagenase injection. The use of local anesthesia for these injections appears to be widespread in the collagenase community, despite not being included in the official FDA protocol.

The FDA prescribes a single dose of collagenase per cord, but following the prescribed dosing instructions results in the waste of a small amount of the medication in the single-use vial. It is now the authors' common practice to use *all* the medication in the vial. In patients with a single cord, the medication can be distributed along a longer length of the cord, for more complete cord dissolution. Especially thick cords or "Y"-shaped junctures where 2 cords join can benefit from use of this little bit of extra medication. If no other uses are in evidence, it can be used to potentially soften heavy palmar nodules present in these patients. Once again, this is an off-label use of the product, but one currently being used by many practitioners.

Although collagenase is now approved for use in 2 cords at once, using 2 vials of the drug, the authors have found that very narrow cords only need a partial dose to effectively cause cord rupture; patients with very narrow cords may be able to achieve dissolution of more than one cord using a single vial of the medication. Alternatively, patients with very narrow cords can be counseled toward needle aponeurotomy, obviating collagenase altogether.

The technique of the injection itself warrants additional notes. Before injection of any local anesthesia, it is the authors' practice to carefully mark out the existing cords with a dotted line using a skin marker. The cords and nodules are marked along their most prominent, palpable aspects, so that the surgeon can get a mental picture of the cord position or positions and the trajectory the injection or injections must take (**Fig. 3**A). It is also helpful to mark the exact sites for injection, because this is where the small amount of local anesthetic will be instilled. During the collagenase injection, the surgeon's nondominant hand is occupied with the passive extension of the patient's involved digits, as well as careful palpation to detect the cords during the process of the injection, which is administered with the dominant hand (**Fig. 3**B, C).[1] The injection should be into the firm, nonyielding tissue of the cord/nodule; if the injection proceeds easily, then the needle is likely missing the cord entirely. A successful injection should be difficult, which of course makes it all the more challenging to maintain gentle, firm pressure on the syringe plunger while not displacing the needle tip from the intended target.

Following injection, the patient is placed in a generously padded dressing: the bulk of the dressing is often surprising to the patient. The authors explain to the patient that they are likely to get quite sore, swollen, and bruised, and that this

padded bandage will typically feel pretty good after a few hours. They are invited to remove the dressing that evening or the following day at their discretion. The authors typically advise the use of over-the-counter pain remedies if needed for this procedure; it is rare to have a patient request additional medication.

One week later, on the day of the manipulation, the patient is given a generous field anesthetic block of the area, enough to completely infiltrate ("tumesce") the region. After allowing about 10 minutes for the block to have maximum effect, the finger in question is gently pulled toward extension to confirm a good local anesthetic block. Once confirmed, the manipulation proceeds in earnest.

After preparing the skin with an alcohol swab, the skin in the area of the cord is massaged in a circular motion using sterile gauze. The goal of this maneuver is to help separate the underlying cord from the skin, which might help decrease the chance of skin tear once the cord eventually ruptures. After a thorough massage to "soften" the area, the patient's wrist is placed in moderate flexion (taking all tension off the flexor tendons), and the joints are stretched into extension. First, the MCP and PIP are done in isolation, then in unison, until all potential cords have ruptured or "popped." Even when cord rupture appears to be complete, the authors often find that sustained passive extension on the finger, combined with direct fingertip pressure over the course of the cord, leads to additional small "pops" as small interconnections of the fascia are disrupted. Web space and thenar cords may require more innovative stretching procedures to completely disrupt these contractures. After manipulation is complete, the patient is asked to perform composite finger flexion to confirm all flexor tendons are intact.

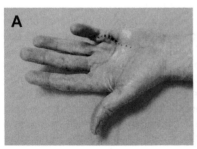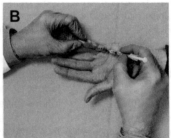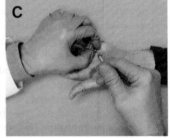

Fig. 3. (*A*) Before injection, the course of the palpable cords is marked with a dotted line. Additional "X" marks are placed over the sites of intended injection. (*B*) As injection proceeds, the nondominant hand maintains passive extension stretch on the digit, keeping the cords taut. (*C*) While maintaining stretch on the digit with the ulnar digits of the nondominant hand, the surgeon can still palpate the cord with the index and thumb, increasing precision of injection.

If a skin tear occurs during manipulation, it often happens at the site of a skin blister ("blood blister"). These skin blisters are especially common when injecting a superficial cord, because some of the collagenase likely has an effect on the dermis itself (**Fig. 4**). Preparing the skin before manipulation can reduce bacterial contamination of these wounds, and keeping a clean gauze pad over the area during the manipulation can reduce the chance of an unexpected spray of blood from a broken blister or skin tear. Skin tears are treated with local wound care; the authors' preference is to dress with antibiotic ointment, nonstick gauze, and a light outer dressing. The dressing is changed at least daily until healing is complete, usually tears heal within 3 to 4 weeks.

After manipulation, and following dressing of any wounds, the patient is referred to hand therapy for creation of a protective extension splint. Patients are instructed to wear this at night, but to leave it off during the day to encourage participation of the hand in daily activities. New problems with stiffness have not been noted with this approach. The hand therapist may work with the patient to help reduce swelling, monitor wound healing, and treat residual contractures with stretching and splinting as needed.

In the authors' experience, most patients obtain significant improvements with one round of collagenase treatment. If successive rounds are indicated, they are scheduled at least 4 weeks apart. Recurrences are reevaluated according to the parameters above, and shared decision making is used to determine the best course of action. Patients with rapid recurrence after collagenase treatment are counseled to consider fasciectomy in the future, because that procedure should provide a more long-lasting result.

INTERVENTION: OPERATIVE

With innovation in nonoperative treatment of Dupuytren contracture, the rate of surgical treatment of this condition has decreased. However, fasciectomy is indicated for patients with PIP joint contracture that may involve multiple cords, such as lateral cord, spiral cord, and central cord. Also, the retrovascular cord that can cause distal interphalangeal joint (DIP) contracture is difficult to be treated by either collagenase or needle aponeurotomy, because the digital neurovascular bundles are intimately attached to the cord. In addition, the chronic PIP contracture requires volar capsulotomy to restore full extension of the PIP joint.

The conduct of an open fasciectomy requires a clear understanding of the neurovascular bundles in relationship to the cords that may tend to displace the neurovascular bundle medially. In many situations, trapped neurovascular bundles under the cord causes the neurovascular bundle to meander along the digit to be displaced both laterally and medially.

There are several essential features for fasciectomy that require consideration:

1. Use sharp dissections with fresh scalpel blades to limit the trauma to the digit. A fresh, sharp no. 15 blade provides efficiency in elevating the skin flaps by the "push" movement around the cords. Dissecting with a knife blade requires tactile sensibility to separate the tough, unyielding cords from the underlying neurovascular bundle that is soft in consistency. It requires some training to feel the difference of the textures between the contracted cord and the underlying softer neurovascular bundle.
2. Be cognizant that occasionally the scrub assistant may exchange the blade without

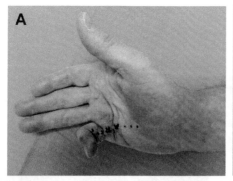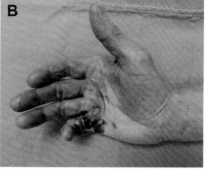

Fig. 4. (*A*) A 61-year-old patient with right small finger Dupuytren contracture, with significant tethering and shortening of the skin, marked for collagenase injection. (*B*) During manipulation, a skin tear occurred at the base of the small finger. In the authors' experience, these uniformly heal within 3 to 4 weeks with local wound care.

informing the surgeon. The essence of the sharp dissection is the feel of the blade against the cords. Changing of the blades can cause neurovascular bundle injury because one may push too hard with a sharper blade that may provide a different perception of the cord texture.

3. In finding the neurovascular bundle, traditional teaching is to dissect out the neurovascular bundles proximally. However, because the neurovascular bundle proximally at the level of the A1 pulley is quite deep, rough soft tissue spreading using scissors can cause increased scarring that limits postoperative rehabilitation and healing. The neurovascular bundle should be found in the "soft spot" of the PIP joint where it is located rather superficially. When the cords encase the PIP joint, the approach to identify the soft spot at the proximal phalanx is suitable (**Fig. 5**). The neurovascular bundle should be identified first before removing the overlying cord.

4. Another challenge with Dupuytren surgery is the uncertainty with the anatomy of the surrounding structures. A surgeon who tends to use scissors in blunt dissection not only causes neurapraxia, but may contuse the vessel in addition to causing tissue trauma by aggressive spreading that tears tissues. The spreading of scissors should be limited to identifying the structures, and the dissection of the cord is performed using a sharp, fresh no. 15 blade. The cords are intimately attached to the neurovascular bundle; therefore, it is more efficient and more precise to use blades on the tough unyielding cord that can be displaced from the underlying compressed neurovascular bundle.

5. The retrovascular cord is the main cause of DIP joint contracture. The neurovascular bundle is displaced volarly by the retrovascular cord (**Fig. 6**). Therefore, retracting the neurovascular bundle medially or laterally from the retrovascular cord gives access to excise the retrovascular cord fully.

6. After all of the cords are removed, the PIP joint may still be contracted. An open volar capsulotomy is performed by opening up the A3 pulley and retracting the flexor digitorum profundus tendon and flexor digitorum superficialis tendon to expose the volar plate. Making an incision over the proximal volar plate extending to the volar portion of the collateral ligament should enable the PIP joint to extend fully. There is no need for pinning of the joint in routine cases. However, in severe contracture of the PIP joint, pinning the joint in a fully extended position for 2 weeks after the release is prudent, so that the release of the volar plate and collateral ligament can reconstitute in the lengthened state. This will help achieve better outcomes with the postoperative therapy.

7. In chronic severe contractures of the PIP joint, extension of the PIP joint may cause neurovascular bundle stretching. If the color of the distal pulp is pale with full extension of the PIP joint, one needs to flex the PIP joint to a certain point for the vascularity to be restored to the fingertip. Then, the PIP joint can be pinned in that position. At a later time, the therapist can stretch out the PIP joint once the finger is acclimated to the stretching of the joint. Never leave the operating room with an ischemic fingertip.

8. For closure with Z-plasties, a 60° Z-plasty is made at the base of the finger by breaking up the linear incision down the midline of the digit (**Fig. 7**). The position of the skin flap needs to

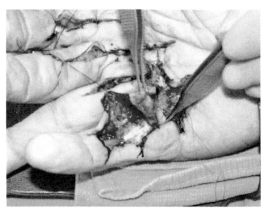

Fig. 5. If the cords encase the PIP joint, the separation of the neurovascular bundle from the cord is performed in the "soft spot" along the proximal phalanx, and then the central cord is released.

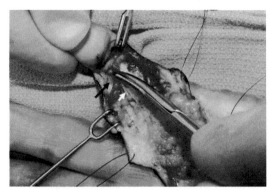

Fig. 6. The retrovascular cord (*black arrow*) lies deep to the neurovascular bundle (*white arrow*).

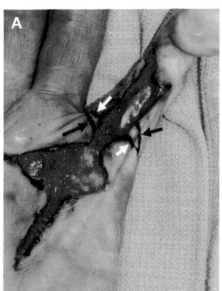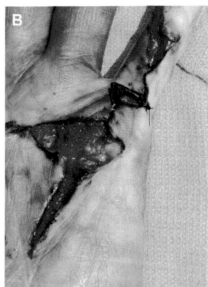

Fig. 7. A Z-plasty is created at the base of the little finger. (*A*) A transverse reference line is made first (*white arrows*), followed by the incision lines (*black arrows*) above and below those marks. (*B*) The 60° Z-plasty lengthens the linear incision.

be designed by recognizing that the neurovascular bundle is under the flap. The Z-plasty causes tension at the base of the finger that can compress the neurovascular bundles. With swelling after surgery, the Z-plasty may be a compression area that causes vascular problems. Therefore, one should not make the Z-plasty overly tight.

The sutures should be removed in about 2 weeks, and the patient is asked to continue to stretch the finger passively for the next 6 months. The patient should wear a finger splint at night to prevent relaxation of the finger, causing flexion contracture when the patient awakes. The wound-healing process, including maturation of scar tissue, should subside in approximately 6 months. Therefore, during this critical period, the patient needs to be informed to be actively involved in stretching the finger with passive extension of the PIP joint. Without this admonition, the patient may simply rely on the therapist to help and not do anything at home. Usually, the authors emphasize to the patients that the stretching needs to be incorporated into the daily routine and built into a habit to constantly stretch the PIP joint with stress-relaxation technique. Stretching of the PIP joint should be done until the skin becomes pale for several minutes, after which time the patient relaxes the finger. This exercise is continued several times a day. This aggressive stretching exercise should prevent recurrent contracture of the finger.

The open fasciectomy procedure is a complex operation. The surgeon has one chance to fix this problem, because revision fasciectomy can lead to several complications, such as neurovascular bundle damage and the inability to fully extend the joint because the tissue in reoperative surgery will feel like concrete. If the Dupuytren contracture recurs, a repeat surgery is often advocated, but it is associated with high risks of creating more scar tissue, the inability to release the contracture fully, as well as potential complications like neurovascular bundle injury. In these situations, fusion of the PIP joint with shortening of the finger can restore finger extension so that the patient can wear a glove in cold climates. In select situations, amputation can also be considered for recurrent Dupuytren contracture.

The authors present tips for surgery of the Dupuytren contracture that can achieve optimal outcomes. Fasciectomy is a rewarding but highly intense and challenging procedure because the anatomy of the neurovascular bundles and the cords are not the same for every patient. However, by adhering to the described principles, surgeons can achieve efficient conduct of the surgical procedure such that even with 3 fingers being operated, one can limit tourniquet time to less than 2 hours. Tourniquet time needs to be within 2 hours because swelling following reperfusion of the fingers can cause an exuberant amount of edema, leading to inability to close all the wounds. The wound closure needs to be meticulous, but there is no need to be airtight. As long as the skin flaps touch each other without folding inwards, the wounds will heal. Small openings over the palm can be treated with dressing changes, which eventually will contract and close uneventfully.

TECHNIQUE: FASCIECTOMY

The patient is placed on an arm board with a tourniquet placed on the upper arm. A lead hand is used to retract and stabilize the fingers. The authors use a longitudinal incision over the palmar surface of the finger with an extended V incision of the level of the PIP joint and a transverse incision over the palmar crease (**Fig. 8**). At closure, the authors make a 60° Z-plasty at the base of the finger to break up the linear incision. A no. 15 blade is used to elevate the skin flaps over the palm, proceeding to elevating the skin flaps over the proximal phalanx and a V extension distally. In the elevation of the skin flap at the level of the dermis, one needs to continue to check on both sides of the skin flap to be sure not to buttonhole the skin flap. Skin laceration will cause sloughing because of disruption of blood supply to the dermal plexus.

After the skin flap is raised, the "soft spot" is found at the level of the PIP joint or any point along the proximal phalanx.[2] The neurovascular bundle is then identified, and the no. 15 blade is used to tease out the neurovascular bundle from the surrounding cords gently. Scissors can be used judiciously, not in the rough spreading format, but gentle spreading to simply identify the neurovascular bundle. At no point should the cords or the tissue around the neurovascular bundle be ripped. The rough handling of soft tissue can cause a significant amount of scarring that limits the recovery

after the surgery. Because cords displace the neurovascular bundle medially and many times compresses the neurovascular bundle, it is essential to find neurovascular bundles both proximally and distally to the cords so that one can trace the path of the neurovascular bundles. In many cases, the neurovascular bundle will be pushed medially by the spiral cords (**Fig. 9**).

When one finds the neurovascular bundle, the cord can be gently released with pushing motion of a sharp no. 15 blade. Once the cord with a gritty feeling is released, the knife will encounter a soft area under the cord that will represent the neurovascular bundle. "Keep your enemy close" is an absolute essential for surgery of the Dupuytren contracture, because the blade continues to trace the neurovascular bundle, keeping the neurovascular bundle close to the blade, and dissect the cord away from the neurovascular bundle, by recognizing the torturous path of the neurovascular bundle.

In a severe contracture, there is a temptation to release a contracted central cord to promote the extension of the finger so that dissection can be easier. However, this is treacherous because one will not be able to predict where the neurovascular bundle lies in relationship to the central cord. Therefore, once one has found the path of the neurovascular bundle on either side of the finger, the central cord can be released sharply with a no. 15 blade to extend the finger, which gives easier access to the dissection.

The neurovascular bundle is traced from the PIP joint proximally so that the bundle can be retracted laterally. Then, the bundle is traced distally. The retrovascular cord that causes flexion of the DIP joint is now identified. Once the neurovascular bundle is fully displayed, then, all cords including the retrovascular cord, lateral cord, spiral cord, and central cord can be excised sharply with a

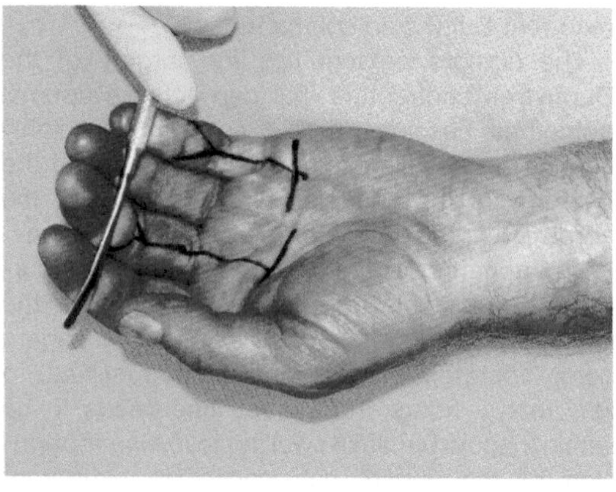

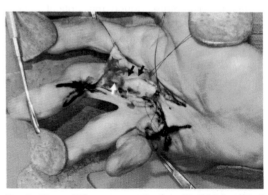

Fig. 8. The authors use a longitudinal incision with a "V" extension at the level of the PIP joint and a transverse incision over the palmar crease.

Fig. 9. The radial neurovascular bundle (*black arrows*) is pushed medially (ulnarly) by the spiral cord (*white arrow*).

no. 15 blade over the pulley system. One should be careful not to resect the pulleys in continuity with the overlying cords.

At the level of the palm, one may encounter the natatory cords that cause adduction of fingers toward each other. During excision of the natatory cords, one should not violate the fat pad at the palm between the fingers because essential perforating vessels to the palmar skin are located between the fingers (**Fig. 10**). At the level of the proximal palm, the neurovascular bundles lie under the transverse palmar fascia (**Fig. 11**). The transverse fibers of the palmar aponeurosis are noted in the literature not involved with Dupuytren disease and can be left in place to protect the underlying neurovascular bundle. Thus, the central cord over the transverse fibers can be removed without concern for a nerve injury, if the transverse fibers are left intact. However, when the transverse fibers are quite thick, removal of the offending contracted cords can be performed judiciously.

After the cords are removed, the fingers should be fully extended. If there is residual DIP contracture, the retrovascular cord dorsal to the DIP joint should be fully resected. Occasionally, the PIP joint may still be contracted. In this situation, the authors incise the volar plate with a sweeping motion around the joint to release the fanlike portion of the collateral ligament. Gentle passive extension of the finger will fully extend the PIP joint by detaching the residual contracted fibers of the collateral ligament. If one feels the PIP joint pop in and out of the joint, this is usually the result of the collateral ligaments not fully released and popping over the condyles. In those situations, the volar portion of the collateral ligament needs to be incised a little more so that the patient can have the smooth extension of the PIP joint.

A 60° Z-plasty is made by first making a transverse mark over the base of the finger, and above and below the mark one would design a 60° Z-plasty. One should be cognizant of the

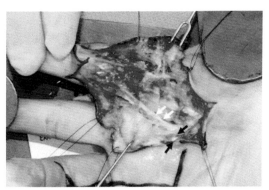

Fig. 11. Because the transverse palmar aponeurosis (*black arrows*) is located superficial to the neurovascular bundles (*white arrows*), the cord over the transverse fibers can be removed without concern for a nerve injury.

underlying neurovascular bundle so that they are not disturbed, and the flaps are sutured in place using 4-0 nylon sutures. The patient's fingers are then fully extended, and the tourniquet is released.

If the finger takes more than a minute to perfuse with full extension of the PIP joint, the PIP joint needs to be flexed, and the perfusion of the fingertip will restore immediately. In these situations, the joint can be pinned in the more flexed posture. The pin can be removed after about 2 weeks at the time of the suture removal, and then stretching exercises can be initiated to restore motion. At no point should a finger be kept in a fully extended posture when the fingertip is pale. Never leave the operating room with a pale finger.

All the wounds are closed using 4-0 nylon suture. Occasionally, there may be difficulties in closing the palm, because of apparent retraction or shortening of the skin due to the disease process. In many cases, the authors have been surprised that release of the convoluted skin leads to enough "stretching" of the skin so that the skin is loose in almost every case. However, if skin closure is a problem over the palm, one can leave small wounds open that can be treated with dressing changes, and invariably the palmar skin will heal quite nicely. All the finger wounds should be able to be closed primarily and then placed in a volar splint; the patient should return to the clinic in about 1 week for a wound check.

All the sutures should be removed in about 2 weeks. The patient should initiate scar massage exercises as aggressively as possible and continue to extend the fingers in concert with a therapist. These stretching exercises of the fingers need to be performed many times a day to prevent any recurrence for the next 6 months.

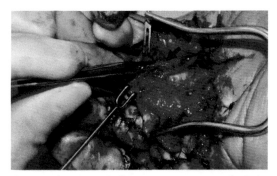

Fig. 10. The arrow indicates a natatory cord of the fourth web space.

A   **B**

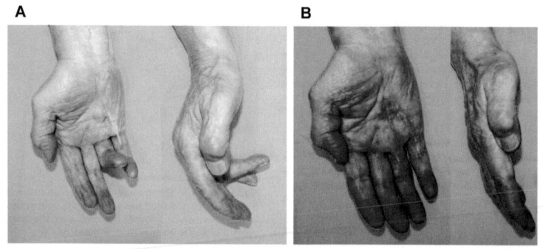

Fig. 12. The postoperative progress after a fasciectomy performed on a right hand. (*A*) Preoperative photographs of the patient's hand. (*B*) The patient gained full extension of the affected fingers 6 weeks after the fasciectomy.

At 6 weeks when the patient returns to the clinic, the wound will have healed, and the patient should have full extension of the finger with occasional residual contracture depending on how severe the contractures are before surgery (**Fig. 12**).

The conduct of a sharp dissection with meticulous respect for the neurovascular bundles and precise identification of all the structures during surgery as well as aggressive patient motivated therapy assures a predictably good outcome of a fasciectomy procedure with relatively few complications.

SUMMARY

Whether by use of needles or scalpels, treatment of patients with Dupuytren disease requires a detailed knowledge of anatomy, careful technique, and attention to detail. As with any complex disease with many treatment options, and no long-lasting "cure," patient-centered care and shared decision-making are of paramount importance.

REFERENCES

1. Giladi AM, Haase SC. Enzymatic treatment with collagenase clostridium histolyticum injection. In: Chung KC, editor. Operative techniques: hand and wrist surgery. 3rd edition. Philadelphia: Elsevier, Inc; 2017. p. 741–6.

2. Giladi AM, Chung KC. Limited open fasciectomy for dupuytren contracture. In: Chung KC, editor. Operative techniques: hand and wrist surgery. 3rd edition. Philadelphia: Elsevier, Inc; 2017. p. 750–6.

Moving?

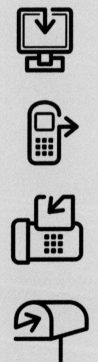